CZ

Targeting Autism

D0965040

Targeting Autism

WHAT WE KNOW, DON'T KNOW, AND CAN DO TO HELP YOUNG CHILDREN WITH AUTISM AND RELATED DISORDERS

Updated Edition

SHIRLEY COHEN

UNIVERSITY OF CALIFORNIA PRESS
Berkeley   Los Angeles   London

University of California Press
Berkeley and Los Angeles, California

University of California Press, Ltd.
London, England

© 1998 by
Shirley Cohen

Updated Edition, 2002

Library of Congress Cataloging-in-Publication Data

Cohen, Shirley.
    Targeting autism : what we know, don't know, and can do to help
young children with autism and related disorders / Shirley Cohen.—
Updated ed.
        p.   cm.
    Includes bibliographical references and index.
    ISBN 0-520-23480-4 (alk. paper)
    1. Autism in children. I. Title.
RJ506.A9 C63   2002
618.92'8982—dc21   2002022505

Printed in the United States of America

10   09   08   07   06   05   04   03   02

9   8   7   6   5   4   3   2   1

To the real Nellie and Sean, wherever they may be

Contents

Acknowledgments

I wish to thank parents and other family members who shared their stories with me; the adults with autism who shared their experiences through presentations, written accounts, and personal encounters; the children with autism who were my teachers; the professionals who allowed me to observe their intervention programs and answered my questions; and the friends who supported my efforts to write this book.

Two friends in particular have my gratitude. Joan Chaplan was my cheerleader and unofficial preliminary editor from the book's conception. Her feedback helped me stay on track most of the time and recognize when I had strayed. Nicholas Anastasiow, well known in the field of special education for many years, praised my efforts enthusiastically even as he pinpointed ideas in need of clearer presentation. I am lucky to have such supportive friends. I also thank Theresa Flannery, who took time from her hectic schedule of parenting, working, and engaging in advocacy to give me a parent's view of my first efforts in writing several chapters of this book; and Kenneth Pomeranz—professor, parent, and advocate—who gave me extensive feedback on the completed manuscript. Final thanks must go to Stanley Holwitz of the University of California Press, who provided support for this book throughout the process of its preparation.

Prologue to the Updated Edition

Targeting Autism presents a comprehensive first excursion into the world of autism. This book was largely written in 1996, with additions and modifications made in the first half of 1997. Although much has remained the same, significant developments have taken place in the world of autism since then. A few of the changes have had immediate impact upon the lives of young children with autism and their families. Other events had no direct effect immediately but are, nonetheless, exciting because of their potential for improving lives in the future. This prologue and the updated appendix of resources include information about new developments and new ways of thinking that have recently modified the map of the world of autism or may do so in the near future.

The prologue is organized into three parts to parallel the three sections of the book. Those readers who are new to the field of autism should read chapter 1 before continuing with this prologue so as to familiarize themselves with basic concepts and terminology, which are presented in that chapter. Some readers may find it useful to alternate between the parts of the book and the sections of the prologue that add new ideas to those sections.

PART ONE

Autism has not changed, but awareness of it has. Parents of young children with autism have helped it change—parents active in national, state, and local advocacy groups; parents like football players Doug Flutie and Dan Marino, who have used their name recognition to raise awareness and money; parents in the film community who have used their access to important audiences to press for research funds; parents who are physicians and researchers and have turned their energies toward autism. Autism has insinuated itself into many families from all walks of life, and families have greatly strengthened the fight against it. Autism awareness rallies in Washington and designation of autism awareness months in the states are new phenomena characteristic of the beginning of the twenty-first century.

Autism has not changed, but there has been a shift in the way we commonly refer to the group of disorders associated with this term. "Pervasive developmental disorders" is still the category label used in the *Diagnostic and Statistical Manual* of the American Psychiatric Association; however, the terms "autistic spectrum disorder" and "autism spectrum disorders" are being used increasingly in its place. These terms have the benefit of being easier for parents and other nonspecialists to understand; they also more clearly communicate the idea that autism is not a neatly packaged unitary disorder.

Autism has not changed, but the autistic spectrum disorder that has moved from the background to share the foreground with autistic disorder is Asperger's syndrome. Until recently this diagnostic label was used largely for older children and adolescents who had often not been identified in early childhood as having a pervasive developmental disorder. Today, the diagnosis of Asperger's syndrome is being made with greater frequency during the preschool and early school years. To some extent it has displaced the label "pervasive developmental disorder not otherwise specified" (PDD-NOS) for children over four or five years of age who communicate verbally and don't meet the more stringent criteria for autistic disorder.

Is Autism Becoming More Common?

Autism has not changed, but the reported prevalence of autism has in-creased dramatically during the past few years, and references have been made to an autism explosion. A decade ago the accepted rate of oc-currence was 4 or 5 per 10,000. In 1996 the more widely accepted rate was 10 to 15 per 10,000. Today a widely accepted figure is 1 per 500, and estimates like 1 per 150 to 200 for the full spectrum are also beginning to appear. The largest reported increase in prevalence has occurred in the milder forms of autistic spectrum disorders, with some researchers re-porting figures as high as 3 or more per 1,000 for Asperger's syndrome alone.

Something real has obviously been happening to bring about such a large increase in the reported prevalence of autistic spectrum disorders. The question still to be resolved is how much of this increase is a result of earlier identification and a greater willingness by physicians and psy-chologists to use diagnostic labels on the autistic spectrum with young children, and how much of it represents a true increase in prevalence. The large increase in Asperger's syndrome in particular may reflect more familiarity with this diagnostic label and better identification. Of course, it may also reflect a substantial increase in the number of chil-dren with milder versions of autism. The Children's Health Act of 2000 directed the Department of Health and Human Services to study this question of prevalence through the establishment of centers on the epi-demiology of autism.

Etiology: The Search Continues

Autism has not changed, but has there been a change in its etiology? If autistic spectrum disorders are, in fact, more common today than they were in earlier decades, what is causing this? The answer presented most frequently during the past few years by parents is vaccines. Why vaccines? The hypothesized genetic basis of autism—the prevalent view of the etiology of autism when the numbers of young children with autism began to increase dramatically—did not seem adequate to account for this phenomenon. What many parents began to notice was a close connection in time between the administration of a triple vaccine for measles, mumps, rubella (MMR) when their children were twelve to fifteen months old and a striking behavioral deterioration in their babies. The medical community explained this association as a noncausal coincidence in time, but many parents did not accept this answer, and a few physicians began to support their view.

Vaccines had long been recognized as causing problems in a tiny fraction of young children, but the number of children involved was considered so low and the benefits of vaccines so imposing that this problem received only limited attention from the medical community. Before the MMR vaccine became the focus of controversy in regard to autism the pertussis toxin in the DPT vaccine was identified as posing a risk of brain damage for some young children, and action was taken to produce a safer version of this vaccine. The recently increasing reluctance of parents to subject their babies to the standard schedule of vaccinations has been putting pressure on the medical community to take a closer look at this situation.

Parents and their supporters have raised several questions. Why are multiple vaccines routinely administered to infants on the same day? Why aren't the components of the MMR vaccine available separately? Was the total amount of mercury included until very recently in the vaccines administered to children during the early years safe? The role, if any, that the current heavy schedule of vaccines administered to young children plays in the increasing number of children identified as having autistic spectrum disorders is an issue in serious need of further study.

Perhaps the most encouraging development in the search for the causes of autistic spectrum disorders is the significant expansion of funding for research in this area in recent years. These dollars are coming from the National Institutes of Health; from states like California; and from private donations, some quite large, to organizations or centers dedicated to the mission of identifying the causes of autism and finding ways to vanquish them. Studies that may help us clarify the role of genetic, prenatal, and postnatal factors in the etiology of autistic spectrum disorders are being carried out today at numerous sites across the country.

PART TWO

Yet Another "Miraculous" Treatment

Supposed breakthroughs in treating autism are still appearing. Unfortunately, none has proven to be a major breakthrough for most children with this disorder. Secretin was the best-publicized supposed breakthrough of the late 1990s. This is what we've been waiting for, announced Bernard Rimland, director of the Autism Research Institute in San Diego, with much fanfare in 1998. The reports by Rimland and Victoria Beck, the mother who first convinced a doctor to administer secretin to her three-year-old son and later told the world of his remarkable improvement, sent hundreds of parents scurrying to find a doctor who would administer this substance.

Secretin does appear to have a beneficial effect on the gastrointestinal systems of some autistic children who have significant problems with the functioning of that system. Behavioral improvements were also noted in some of these children, but behavioral improvement is not surprising when chronic physical problems such as diarrhea and its accompanying discomfort are eliminated. Yet a small number of children with autism demonstrated substantial improvements in social interaction and language that appeared to go beyond what might have been expected on the basis of relief from gastrointestinal problems alone.

All the answers about secretin are not yet in. Under the pressure of thousands of individuals with autism being given this substance in off-label use, often at extremely high cost, the National Institutes of Health authorized five studies of secretin around the country. To date, the preponderance of data places secretin in the same category as supposed breakthroughs from earlier years. It may provide significant help to a tiny percentage of children with autism, while having little or no effect upon the functioning of most children with this disorder. More research is needed on the small subset of children who seem to demonstrate improvement after receiving this substance. Such research may have the potential to shed light on one source of autistic characteristics in children.

Loosening the Grip of Autism Through Early Intervention

One answer about the treatment of autistic spectrum disorders that seems quite solid is the importance of early intervention. In order to provide early intervention, children need to be identified at a young age. The early tools for diagnosing autism were not designed for children below age three, and clinicians were generally reluctant to use that label with children below this age. However, recently substantial attention has been devoted to ways of identifying autism in infants and toddlers, and many children are now identified as having autistic spectrum disorders at two years of age or even earlier.

The American Academy of Neurology and the Child Neurology Society recently produced practice parameters for the screening and diagnosis of autism. These guidelines call for "Routine Developmental Surveillance and Screening Specifically for Autism" with all young children, first to identify children at risk for all types of atypical development and then to identify children specifically at risk for autism. The Checklist for Autism in Toddlers (CHAT) is one of the instruments recommended for conducting the screening specifically for autism, with children identified through such screening then being referred for a comprehensive evaluation. This brief and simple procedure was designed to screen large populations of children for autism at about eighteen months of age. A modified version of this screening instrument—the M-CHAT—is currently being tested in a large-scale validation study.

While identification at about eighteen months is a big step toward ensuring early intervention and better outcomes, it is likely that methods of identifying some children with autism at even earlier ages will soon be developed. Several studies of home videotapes made of babies at nine to twelve months of age point to significant differences even at that early age.

Educational Models and Services

Autism hasn't changed, but (good news!) intervention services for young children have. In many parts of the country early intervention services for children under age three with the diagnosis of autism have been expanded substantially. For example, the current New York State Department of Health early intervention guidelines call for a minimum of twenty hours a week of individualized services in behavioral programs. Five years earlier, children under age three generally received about two hours a week of early intervention services in this system.

Applied behavior analysis (ABA) has become widely recognized as an effective intervention approach for many young children with autism. There are significant variations in this approach, and lately parent interest in more naturalistic versions of ABA has increased. This increase probably reflects concerns about the stressfulness and restrictions of discrete trial instruction for very young children as well as some disappointment with the outcomes of ABA intervention programs focused heavily on such instruction. Many of the better ABA programs are now expanding the role of more naturalistic strategies in their approach: increasing their focus on use of new skills in functional situations; incorporating more opportunities for choice and initiation by children throughout the day; and placing more emphasis on social interactive skills.

Inclusion is the current educational password for students with special needs and the goal of most parents of young children with autistic spectrum disorders. However, many parents of children with autistic spectrum disorders are fighting for another option for their school-age children. To these parents inclusion does not address some of the central needs of their children. Often this is so because the conditions that make successful inclusion possible are not present—support from administrators; adequate training and ongoing assistance from skilled specialists for mainstream teachers; carefully selected and trained assistant teachers; one-to-one direct instruction as needed; and appropriate functional behavioral assessments and plans. In other cases the nature or intensity of a child's needs leads parents to believe that a special program would be more appropriate.

Surprisingly, some of the children whose parents are opting for special programs are children with Asperger's syndrome. Because these children are generally bright and highly verbal, the extent of their disability is often not recognized, and the mainstream does not provide the help they desperately need in understanding and dealing with novel or socially demanding situations.

PART THREE

Outcomes: New and Awaited Data

The 47 percent recovery rate reported by Ivar Lovaas in 1987 helped to ignite a stampede for ABA services among parents, although many professionals questioned his outcome data on multiple grounds. While Lovaas responded to these criticisms vigorously, it was his replication project, supported by funds from the National Institute of Mental Health, that had the potential to silence his critics. The results of this study were, therefore, awaited with great interest, and are still being awaited.

In the meantime, a report of children receiving services from the UCLA Young Autism Project between 1989 and 1992 was recently published by Smith and others. The children in this study received an average of twenty-five hours of services. Only two of the fifteen children met the criteria for "best outcome" used in earlier studies, namely placement in general education classes without special education services and an IQ greater than 85. This is a 13 percent "recovery" rate, very different from the initially reported rate of 47 percent. Is the reduction in hours from forty to twenty-five a sufficient explanation for this poorer outcome? We await the results of the multi-site Young Autism Project for clarification.

In the meantime other programs using various types of ABA models have reported on outcomes. The percentage of children able to function in general education classes with little or no support after leaving these

ABA programs ranges from about 15 percent to about 50 percent (Handleman and Harris 2001). We need to learn more about why some of these programs appear to have substantially better outcomes than do others.

Still Moving Toward Better Answers

The past few years have been relatively good ones for the autism community. Awareness of autism has expanded greatly. Research funds have increased substantially. Earlier identification is now possible and common. Early intervention services have become more intensive, and there has been an expansion of programs for preschoolers. Moreover, more children with autism have developed functional language by the time they enter programs for school-age children (i.e., before age five or six) than has ever been the case in the past.

While we continue to strive for the means to prevent and/or cure autism, more can be accomplished to improve lives. Education still needs to become better. Special education teachers need to know more about how to work productively with children who have autistic spectrum disorders; so, too, do mainstream teachers; and school systems must begin to provide better supports for inclusion of these children and adolescents.

Awareness is a first step. Research, treatment, acceptance, and inclusion are other steps that must be pursued with vigor.

Preface

In late 1993 I received a telephone call at my college office from the mother of a two-year-old boy recently diagnosed as autistic. She was looking for students to work with her son in an in-home behavioral treatment program. I promised to post a notice on the "Jobs" bulletin board of the Department of Special Education. Two more mothers called me for the same purpose a short time after that, and the department chairperson also received a couple of such calls. I asked the mothers with whom I spoke what had made them choose this type of intervention and whether they had looked into other types of approaches or programs. They referred me, sometimes angrily, to a book written by Catherine Maurice, the mother of two autistic children who had "recovered" through an in-home behavioral program designed by O. Ivar Lovaas, a professor at the University of California, Los Angeles. The Lovaas treatment model was not new. Not only had I read his 1981 manual for this approach (*Teaching Developmentally Disabled Children: The ME Book*) about ten years earlier, but I had been dismayed by aspects of his approach. Yet something appeared to be happening that I wanted to understand. I read Catherine Maurice's book and—more than thirty

years after my intensive involvement with autistic children—was drawn
back into the world of autism.

Two autistic children I fervently wanted to help, but couldn't, haunt my
memory. I was a young teacher filled with energy, a sense of mission,
and faith in my own competence and I felt particularly drawn to children who needed special attention and assistance. In 1959 I fell in love
with a group of six- and seven-year-olds at a treatment and research
center for children who were at that time categorized as having childhood schizophrenia or childhood psychosis. Today, almost all those children would be labeled autistic. Some of the children at this center were
helped considerably and went on to enter mainstream education classes;
others showed moderate improvement and went on to special education
classes in public schools; a few showed very little improvement and
were placed in residential treatment centers for adolescents or in institutions. The two students who have haunted my memory these many
years were children I didn't help enough. Could there now really be a
way to help children like Nellie and Sean*? I decided to find out.

The father of an adolescent with autism joked to his audience of parents and professionals at a conference on autism: We parents know why
we're here; we had no choice. But sometimes we wonder about you
professionals. The special education teacher sitting next to me answered
for both of us: Autistic children get into your system and stay there.

This book is the story of autism as I put it together from the vantage
point of over thirty years of professional focus on the education of
young children with disabilities, including an intensive reimmersion
into the study of autism in recent years. This book is not an exhaustive
reference or detailed manual. It is to serve as a sort of road map of the
world of autism for parents, educators, other clinical personnel, and students. For families this book attempts to offer a broader framework and
a richer context of experiences than do the biographical case studies

*I changed the names of individuals with autism and some details about them, unless
the published literature identified them.

written by parents of autistic children. For professionals and students this book attempts to convey the challenge and fascination of autism, while also presenting the best current data and thinking on the subject.

Many stories punctuate the book. Narrative approaches have renewed stature in teaching and learning as a way of clarifying issues, putting behavior into the human context, and enriching communication about behavior. Parents, individuals with autism, and professionals use narrative to share with others what they experienced and learned. While a single narrative may have restricted value, multiple narratives on the same subject, including biographies, case studies, and story fragments, point to important themes in defining problems and understanding dynamics.

The mysterious code of autism remains unbroken, but we now have tools that may loosen its bonds and enable many individuals with autism to emerge into a common life space with the people significant to them. We are also coming much closer to deciphering the code that turns the lives of some children into chaos and spreads havoc and despair throughout their families. This book highlights what we know, what we don't know, what we can do, what controversies exist, and what promising leads may help us achieve the goals of understanding autism and eliminating its devastating effects on the development of children.

part one What Is Autism?

1 Meeting Autism

There she moved, every day, among us but not of us,

acquiescent when we approached, untouched when

we retreated, serene, detached. . . . Existing among

us, she had her being elsewhere.

(Park 1982, 12)

I visit the home of parents I recently met. Their five-year-old son is standing on his head on the couch. I go up to him, turn my head to the side, and say, "Hello, Kenneth." "Hello, Kenneth," he echoes.

I enter a room at a hotel where an informal meeting is taking place. As soon as I step through the doorway, a handsome, nicely dressed young man of perhaps seventeen walks up to me and tells me his name. The following exchange then takes place.

"What is your name?"

"Shirley."

"What is your sister's name?"

"Which sister?"

"How many sisters do you have?"

"Two."

"What are their names?"

"Paula and Sandy."

3

"What is your brother's name?"

"How do you know I have a brother?"

After faltering for a second he continues, "You don't have a brother?"

His attention then immediately shifts to the person who entered the room after me, and the same questioning routine begins again.

I am at a national conference on autism. Walter, a man perhaps in his mid-twenties, draws my attention. He claps loudly when anyone is introduced, and as he does so his mouth opens, his head moves from side to side, and his eyes appear to focus at a point near the ceiling. Walter and his mother are sitting only a few feet from the bluegrass band that is to play at the conference reception. As soon as the loud and lively music starts, Walter's hands begin to twist rapidly in arcs before him, the right one clockwise, the left counterclockwise. He keeps clasping his hands together, whether to stop their movement or to clap I don't know, but his hands keep breaking loose. His head turns faster and faster, keeping time with both his hands and the music. When the music ends, Walter's movements slow to a stop. He looks at the ceiling briefly and then sits quietly.

A woman who has a Ph.D. is making a presentation: Temple Grandin has written two books about herself as well as numerous articles on autism. She is also the subject of an intensive case study in the book *An Anthropologist on Mars* by the neurologist Oliver Sacks. Temple Grandin is a person with autism.

We glimpse here a few of the many faces of autism. One of the most striking aspects of the condition (or conditions) labeled "autism" is its variability. What then do people called autistic have in common? What does that term autism mean if it encompasses such heterogeneity? What is the concept behind the label? To answer this question we need to look across several perspectives—those of researchers, clinicians, parents, and adults with autism. We can begin by studying the "bible" of diagnostic categories and labels, the American Psychiatric Association's *Diagnostic and Statistical Manual of Mental Disorders* (DSM-IV), now in its fourth edition.

Autism is classified by DSM-IV as a pervasive developmental disorder, a term meant to indicate "severe and pervasive impairment in several areas of development: reciprocal social interaction skills, communication skills, or the presence of stereotyped behavior, interests, and activities" (APA 1994, 65). Let's look at what autism may mean through examples provided by parents.

Qualitative impairment in social interaction. Catherine Maurice describes the social isolation of her infant daughter.

> Anne-Marie was not shy: she was largely oblivious to people, and would sometimes actually avoid them, including, a lot of the time, her own mother. She drifted toward solitary spaces: the corners of a room, behind the curtains, behind the armchair. If I was somewhere else in the apartment, she never sought me out. . . .
>
> Worst of all, perhaps, was the lack of that primary connection: the sweet steady gazing into one's eyes that we began to see all around us in other toddlers. . . . Sometimes I would catch her gazing in my direction and would start up, eager to respond to her invitation, to meet her look. But her eyes, frighteningly, were focused upon some middle distance, somewhere between me and the wall behind me. She wasn't seeing me at all. She was looking right through me! (Maurice 1993, 31, 33)

Qualitative impairments in communication. Craig Schulze tells us about his son's speech without communication.

> I then enter the room carrying Jordan's dinner. "Put it on the table," he blurts out when he sees his food. It's a remark he's been making four times a day (during meal times and his snack) for over two weeks. He doesn't seem to really care where I put the food since he darts away from me the minute I'm in the room. Like so many of his most recent utterances, this habitual response seems more a ritual than an attempt at communication. It's spoken in a loud monotone with almost no emotion. (Schulze 1993, 105)

Clara Park describes her daughter's language at age two and then at age twenty-three. At age two her daughter used words, but infrequently and not to communicate. "She had no idea of language as a tool that could cause things to happen" (1982, 74). At age twenty-three,

> Anybody who hears Jessy speak more than a word or two realizes that something is wrong. She has learned English as a foreign tongue, though far more slowly, and she still speaks it as a stranger. The more

excited she is about what she has to say, the more her speech deterio-
rates; her attention cannot stretch to cover both what she is saying and
how she is saying it. Pronouns get scrambled: "you" for "I," "she" for
"he," "they" for "we." Articles and tenses are confused or disappear,
verbs lose their inflections or are omitted altogether. (Park 1982, 292)

*Restricted repetitive and stereotyped patterns of behavior, interests, and ac-
tivities.* "We watched him as he rocked his body and spun every round
object he could find," writes Barry Kaufman in describing his not yet
two-year-old son's repetitive behavior (1976, 62). Judy Barron writes of
her infant son:

> He was drawn to odd things. He'd crawl past a brightly colored selec-
> tion of toys to get to the furnace register. Once there he would stick his
> fingers into the slots and watch his fingers move. There was a hole in
> the wooden floor of his bedroom that riveted his attention. He'd put his
> finger into that and wiggle it around for hours. (Barron and Barron
> 1992, 13)

Six-year-old Paul McDonnell became obsessed with light bulbs, his
mother, Jane, wrote.

> His light bulb collection had grown to include not only incandescent
> household light bulbs, but also fluorescent bulbs, black lights, infrared
> and ultraviolet bulbs, and flashcubes: three hundred seventy-two in all.
> He kept many of his light bulbs in a basket by his bed, and every night
> he tried out different bulbs. (McDonnell 1993, 154)

As an adolescent Temple Grandin became fixated on squeeze chutes for
cattle, an obsession that she later transformed into a therapeutic device
to calm herself and others.

All autistic children do not act exactly like the children described
above. Not all are as cut off from people as was Anne-Marie Maurice;
not all have to struggle as hard as did Jessy Park to use language for
communication; and the stereotyped interests of children with autism
vary widely. See Appendix A for the specific combinations of behavioral
indicators that professionals use to arrive at a diagnosis of autism.

"There are, due to a tragic accident of nature, children with autism who
live in society, but who for some as yet ill-understood reasons cannot

profit much from the social stimulation provided by loving and caring parents" (Volkmar 1993, 40). Who are these children? How many are there?

The Autism Society of America (ASA) estimates that there are about 400,000 people in the United States with some form of autism. For years, the generally accepted rate of occurrence was 4–5 per 10,000, although individual studies sometimes reported higher figures. Recent studies have tended to support a higher prevalence rate, and estimates of 10–15 per 10,000 people are now widely accepted. This shift may reflect an actual increase in the prevalence of autism, but an alternate possibility is that it reflects other factors such as better identification and modifications in diagnostic criteria. Autism used to be considered a low-incidence disorder. Now it is referred to as one of the most common childhood conditions within the category of developmental disorders.

"He" is the common personal pronoun in books on autism, but that usage does not reflect gender bias. Autism is largely a male disorder; for every autistic girl there are approximately four autistic boys. And yet girls diagnosed as autistic are generally more severely impaired and have lower IQs. At this time there is no explanation for this gender difference, although it may well reflect genetic mechanisms. Another pervasive developmental disorder, *Rett syndrome* (or *Rett's disorder*), is virtually exclusive to females and shares many features with autism, thus possibly reflecting a common underlying neurobiological factor or factors.

Autism is more common in some families than in most others. Studies have shown that the prevalence of autism among siblings of autistic individuals is substantially higher than in the general population, and the concordance rate for autism in identical twins is much higher than in nonidentical twins; if one identical twin has autism it is likely that the other one does as well. Furthermore, parents with possible (mild) autism have been identified in some families of autistic children. These findings strengthen the hypothesis that at least some forms of autism have a genetic base. Even when no other person in a family has autism, there may be a higher than expected prevalence of cognitive and social impairments that, while less severe than autism, may point to a common genetic base.

Most people, when they have heard anything at all about autism, have a particular image of it that represents only one of the faces of autism. While the full range of variations in autism may not be apparent in early childhood, one difference clearly is: some children with autism appear different almost from birth, while others appear to develop normally for a period of time and then begin to regress. By the time her daughter was one month old, Annabel Stehli (author of *Sound of a Miracle*) was sure that something was wrong. Time only added confirmation. Georgie did not grasp her mother's finger or look at her or smile or snuggle against her when she was being held. Judy Barron reported a similar experience with her son Sean, who never seemed to want to be held, squirming, twisting, and pushing against her as if he felt trapped when she picked him up.

A very different infancy was experienced by other parents of autistic children, one in which the sense of loss was excruciatingly exacerbated by development suddenly halted and then reversed.

> A clear-eyed boy of nineteen months is pointing to the gaily decorated tree in my living room. "Christmas lights, Daddy," he says as he reaches up to touch the bulbs. "This one is green. This one is blue." Jordan goes through all the colors, carefully pointing out the names of each that he touches. From across the room my wife, Jill, beams as she listens to these first words of the season from our first child. . . .
>
> The here-and-now version of the happy toddler is the seven-year-old boy who, on this day alone, has bitten the school bus driver, flung himself on the floor in a fit of rage in the grocery store, spent nearly half an hour tapping toys on his teeth, and occupied himself in his last waking hour flushing the toilet over twenty times. (Schulze 1993, i–ii)

Autism is usually present within the first year of life, but about one-third of the time it appears to have its onset within the second or third year. However, experts have commented, what is taken to be late onset may sometimes reflect delay in detection owing to parental denial or lack of sophistication. There's no question of delayed detection creating a false appearance of late onset in Jordan Schulze's case. His early development was too advanced and its reversal too sharp a contrast. But I think back to something the mother of my student Nellie said to me over thirty years ago. Nellie was doing all right until she went to nursery school, her mother told me, implying that something had happened at nursery school to cause her daughter's autistic behavior. Yet home films viewed by the clinical staff had shown a picture of two-year-old Nellie, before any nursery school experience, hiding behind furniture and people, not looking or smiling at or playing with anyone. A parent trying to account for unexplainable loss.

Why are there such differences in time of onset and the course of development during the first two or three years? The answer to this question will come only when we discover more about the causes of autism.

Perhaps the major factor accounting for the heterogeneity of the population called autistic is the presence or absence of mental retardation. Professionals report that more than half of all children with autism are mentally retarded, but it is often difficult to determine whether a young child with autism is mentally retarded. Aside from the broader issues of the meaning of IQ and the conceptualization of intelligence, how are we to assess intelligence in children who may have no functional speech or any other organized communicative system; who rarely look at people or follow verbal directions or imitate movements?

Occasionally a child will show unusual abilities that seem to give clues to an answer. Some young autistic children are "hyperlexic"—they learn to read at an early age without formal teaching, in spite of a general delay or deviance in language development, although this reading may be largely word naming with little comprehension. Other children may show different kinds of evidence of prodigious rote memory. Astounding abilities in art, music, and calendar calculations have been noted in autistic individuals who otherwise appear to be moderately to severely mentally retarded, and "islets" of competence in such areas as mathematics are common in autistic individuals who otherwise function at a level considered to indicate mild mental retardation. (Sometimes early signs of autism are not recognized because of such islets of competence in the young child.)

IQ in young children does seem to matter in a major way. A performance IQ approaching 70, combined with some functional language by age five, seems to predict a better developmental course for autistic individuals. But autistic children are idiosyncratic; they break all rules. Some autistic children are nonverbal until well beyond age five and are considered to be mentally retarded, and then they begin to communicate and prove everyone wrong. Yet the variability of intelligence among individuals with autism is unquestionable. Some young children with autism make slow and limited progress in learning even with skilled, intensive intervention, while others have gone from treatment programs to challenging educational programs, and on to college studies in mathematics or science.

What distinguishes autism from other pervasive developmental disorders? Young children who do not strictly meet the criteria for autism are often assigned the label *PDD*, which is a shorthand version of the term "pervasive developmental disorder not otherwise specified" (*PDD/NOS*). Essentially what the PDD label indicates is that the child has some of the defining characteristics of autism but not enough of them, or that the child does not have the intensity of symptoms characteristic of autism. Sometimes well-meaning professionals use the term PDD with very young children when they feel that the label "autism" would be premature and they want to protect families from the frightening associations commonly linked to this term. "Autism is the cancer . . . of the developmental disorders," writes a neurologist explaining the reluctance of professionals to use this diagnosis (Rapin 1994, 2), while PDD is presented as a serious, multifaceted problem in development, but one that is not quite as severe as autism. At times the concern that leads to the use of the PDD label can have unintended negative effects, such as leaving parents confused or increasing the difficulty of obtaining intensive early intervention services for the child.

Another reason for use of the PDD label is parents' growing awareness of the importance of early identification of developmental disabilities and the availability of intervention services for young children with disabilities. While it is possible to identify many children with pervasive developmental disorders at eighteen to twenty-four months of age, at such an age the distinction between autism and PDD/NOS is not always clear.

Childhood disintegrative disorder, or Heller's syndrome, is another pervasive developmental disorder, and it has a very poor prognosis. According to DSM-IV, its essential feature is "a marked regression in multiple areas of functioning following a period of at least two years of apparently normal development." The areas affected include language, social skills or adaptive behavior, play, motor skills, and bowel or bladder control; and this condition is "usually associated with severe mental retardation" (APA 1994, 73, 75). There are no known biological markers that can be used to differentiate childhood disintegrative disorder from autism.

Craig Schulze is an educator with a Ph.D. in human development whose son was diagnosed as autistic, but who came to question this label. In his 1993 book Schulze describes the deterioration of his young son—"It is as if he has died from one existence and returned in another form" (42)—and his own fruitless struggle to return Jordan to his first life. "Psychologists, neurologists, self-styled gurus, teachers (American and Japanese), relatives and friends, even our own intuitions had joined in a continuing chorus of 'We Shall Overcome.' Now the harmony is gone, and the tune is flat, and the voices are silent" (147).

As a panelist at the 1995 convention of the Autism Society of America, Schulze questioned whether his son has autism or Heller's syndrome. Undoubtedly, this man was giving voice to despair over his son's meager response to all the efforts focused on him, but he was also raising doubt about the differential diagnosis of autism and another pervasive developmental disorder with a worse prognosis.

Higher functioning autism by another name is one way of thinking about *Asperger's* (or *Asperger*) *syndrome.* Professionals often refer to this condition as a subtype of autism. DSM-IV treats this disorder as a pervasive developmental disorder separate from autism, although the two share some core characteristics, namely severe impairment in social interaction and restricted, repetitive patterns of behavior, interests, and activities. In contrast to autism, Asperger's syndrome is described in DSM-IV as not being marked by severe delays in the development of language, cognition, self-help skills, or curiosity about the environment in childhood (77). Many children diagnosed with Asperger's disorder or syndrome show delayed motor development and have motor clumsiness that is reflected in difficulty developing such skills as riding a bicycle and catching a ball. They may also display awkwardness or oddness in posture and gait (Klin and Volkmar 1995).

The label "Asperger's syndrome" has recently come into wider use in the United States. Children and adolescents who in the past might have been diagnosed as having emotional disturbance or attention-deficit disorder are now sometimes being labeled or relabeled as having Asperger's syndrome. There also appears to be overlap between children and adolescents identified as having Asperger's syndrome and those identified as having schizoid personality or nonverbal learning disabilities. Individuals with Asperger's syndrome are often "loners." Although most show interest in making friends, their attempts to do so are often unsuccessful. Contributing to such failures are long-winded, one-sided "conversations" about their favorite interests, and insensitivity to other people's feelings and nonverbal communications.

Children with Asperger's syndrome often appear eccentric or emotionally disturbed. In spite of good academic performance, these children seem to lack common sense. This problem may be exacerbated in adolescence, as it was in Rita's case. Rita was not identified as needing special education services when she was a child; academically she functioned on grade level. But in adolescence her behavior appeared to become increasingly age-inappropriate and odd. At age eighteen Rita moved to a group home for adults with disabilities, where the staff tried to help her develop skills she would need to live independently and find work. On one of her weekend trips home Rita appeared to be trying to apply some of the skills she had been taught. She entered a fish store and, after a substantial period of consideration, indicated to the proprietor the particular fish she wanted. After the fish had been weighed and she had been given the price, Rita stated that she was now going home to ask her mother if she could buy it.

Many specialists in autism take the position that Asperger's syndrome is a mild variant of autism, part of a continuum or spectrum of autistic disorders involving impairments in social interaction, communication, and imagination along with rigid, repetitive activity preferences.

A higher than expected frequency of Asperger's syndrome has been found in the families of high-functioning individuals with autism, and Oliver Sacks refers to an entire autistic family—the gifted parents and older son with Asperger's syndrome, the younger son with classic autism—who, "between the serious business of life," flapped their arms, jumped on a trampoline, and screamed (1995, 244).

If Asperger's syndrome is another name for high-functioning individuals with autism, the balance within the category of autism is tipped toward individuals with better language and academic achievement or potential. This would have "political" implications; it could influence the kind of behavioral research that is funded and the kinds of treatment and support services developed. A mother addresses this issue in her letter to the *Advocate*, the newsletter of the Autism Society of America. "As a mother of a severely-autistic self-injurious child, I am saddened by the continual neglect of the most severe cases of autism—and the increasingly dangerous glorification of the so-called high-functioning-curable-autistics" (Gilbert 1995, 4).

This mother raises another issue about classification and labeling, one that is not likely to be answerable until the condition that we now call autism is better understood. She questions whether high-functioning autistic individuals should be grouped with other autistic individuals whose behavior and prognosis is quite different. "It is about time that we start separating the primitive autistics who spend the majority of their day smashing their heads into the wall and biting themselves from the ever so interesting savant group that impresses Oprah Winfrey by playing Chopin." But are these really two distinct conditions or groups, or are they different points on a continuum? Do they have the same etiology, or are the underlying factors different, or is it a matter of a single impairment versus that same impairment plus others? What role does the nature of early environmental experience, including planned treatment, play in these differences? The answers to these questions are still unknown.

Questions can also be raised about the differential diagnosis of autism and other disabilities outside the spectrum of pervasive developmental disorders that may mimic the appearance of autism. Labels indicating categories of disability are most useful when all individuals identified by a particular label exhibit the defining characteristics of that category, when there are clear boundaries between categories, and when an individual who fits into one such category will not meet the criteria for another one. Unfortunately, autism eludes this framework. Autism should be viewed as a working label. When more is known about the cause or causes of this disorder, the label autism may be replaced by several labels, or the way in which we think about this syndrome and related developmental disabilities may be dramatically altered.

Landau-Kleffner syndrome is a disorder that may mimic autism in some ways. The outstanding feature of this syndrome is loss of language after a period of normal development, usually of more than two years and sometimes as long as seven years. On March 9, 1995, an ABC news program called *Day One* included a segment on Landau-Kleffner syndrome. For weeks after that segment was shown, Thomas Jefferson University Hospital in Philadelphia was overwhelmed with telephone calls from parents for Gerry Stefanatos, director of the Center for Clinical and Developmental Neurophysiology, who had been featured in the television program. What had mobilized these parents was a rekindling of hope for the children lost to autism of late onset, children who had been developing as normally expected until perhaps sixteen, eighteen, or twenty-two months of age, when their development seemed to change course. Babies stopped using the words they had already acquired, stopped acquiring new words, stopped trying to communicate through smiles or gestures that they wanted to be picked up or played with, stopped snuggling up to their mothers to receive hugs and kisses, and stopped offering any of their own.

What parents heard and saw on the *Day One* program that gave them hope was a boy who had been labeled as autistic, but who was apparently helped to regain his developmental momentum after being rediagnosed as having Landau-Kleffner syndrome and treated for it. At around age two, T. J. Voeltz had "stopped talking and began to disappear" into his own world. His mother was told that there was nothing medicine could do for her son, who had incurable brain damage; she needed to get on with her life. But Kathy Voeltz did not heed these words, and eventually at a conference on autism she heard a speaker say that anyone who knew a child who used to talk should look into Landau-Kleffner syndrome. She did. After testing, her son's diagnosis was changed, and he was treated with the drug ACTH. Two years later, eight-year-old T. J. Voeltz was in a second-grade class. He spoke; he played; he learned. He could do most of the things that a boy his age is expected to do. His parents believe that several months of treatment had given T. J. a second chance at a normal life. It is what thousands of parents of autistic children have dreamed of.

To parents, the saving grace of Landau-Kleffner syndrome is that medication can sometimes reverse its downward course, whereas no medication has been identified as effective in reversing the core features of autism. But we might question whether the steroid treatment used with T. J. did, in fact, cause his recovery: Landau-Kleffner syndrome is an odd condition; fluctuating progression and spontaneous remissions have sometimes been noted by physicians, and only controlled clinical studies will provide a definitive answer to this question. An even more basic issue has to do with the boundary between autism and Landau-Kleffner syndrome: are these totally distinct conditions, or can their boundaries overlap?

Landau-Kleffner syndrome, identified in 1957, has been considered a condition of very low incidence. As of the early 1990s the literature was still referring to "more than 170" reported cases of this syndrome, which is also referred to as acquired epileptic aphasia. Epilepsy is present in Landau-Kleffner syndrome about 70 percent of the time, and abnormalities in brain-wave patterns are central to the diagnosis of this condition. What complicates the differential diagnosis of late-onset autism and Landau-Kleffner syndrome is the fact that children with autism also have higher than normal rates of epilepsy and abnormal electroencephalograms (EEGs). Seizure disorders have been identified in 25–40 percent of individuals with autism by early adulthood, with two peak periods of incidence, one in early childhood and one in adolescence (Lord and Rutter 1994). Furthermore, many children diagnosed with autism have not had EEGs; and even those who have had an EEG may not have had an extended-sleep EEG, which is often essential for detection of the typical pattern of EEG abnormalities in Landau-Kleffner syndrome. Differentiation between autism and Landau-Kleffner syndrome may also be difficult because behavioral disturbances common to autism— for example, resistance to change and withdrawal—are sometimes found in children with Landau-Kleffner syndrome. Thus, it is possible that this condition is more prevalent than previously considered, and that a number of children diagnosed as having autism of late onset meet the criteria for Landau-Kleffner syndrome.

What are the prospects for successful treatment of children with Landau-Kleffner syndrome, and what does "successful treatment" mean in this context? Landau-Kleffner syndrome is usually treated with anti-convulsant medications and ACTH or corticosteroids such as predni-sone. The number of children who have been treated is probably too small to yield a reliable estimate of successful outcomes, however we define such outcomes. The reported outcomes range from complete, dramatic remission of symptoms—including speech loss, poor language comprehension, and abnormal EEGs—to partial recovery with mild lan-guage disorder and continuing cognitive impairment. A surgical proce-dure, multiple subpial transection (brain surgery), has also been avail-able since about 1990 for use in treating this disorder when medication is not effective. Neither treatment is to be undertaken lightly. Steroids have significant negative side effects, and brain surgery always involves serious risk.

Gerry Stefanatos and associates recently used prednisone to treat a six-year-old boy who had experienced severe regression in language and behavior at twenty-two months, and who had been labeled as PDD/NOS. This boy did not have the EEG pattern associated with Landau-Kleffner syndrome, although other signs pointed in that direc-tion. Stefanatos reported that within several weeks the boy's spontane-ous speech and social relatedness had increased significantly.

In some cases, months after apparently successful drug treatment was discontinued, abnormal EEGs and progressive language loss reappeared in children with Landau-Kleffner syndrome but went into remission when treatment was promptly reinstituted. Both the speed and extent of symptom remission appear related to the length of time from the child's first symptoms to the initial treatment, as well as the adequacy of medication dosage and treatment length. Thus, Landau-Kleffner syndrome should be considered whenever a young child presents with what appears to be autism of late onset, and appropriate testing should be implemented to rule out this condition before a diagnosis of autism is confirmed.

Another condition that shares some distinctive features with autism is obsessive-compulsive disorder. The rituals of obsessive-compulsive individuals sometimes cannot be distinguished from the rituals and repetitive, fixed routines often found in children and adults with autism. Jeffrey's father describes his four-year-old son's behavior:

> I went to father's night at my Jeffrey's pre-school. He was playing with a Fisher-Price toy, a schoolhouse, but his play was strange. He stood before the toy, jumped up and down, and flapped his arms as if excited by it. . . . When the jumping stopped, he would put his arms together and wiggle his fingers just above eye level. . . . He did this for 35 minutes. (Rapoport 1989, 29–30)

The description of Jeffrey's stereotyped behavior makes it easy to begin thinking of autism, but Jeffrey did not have the severe difficulties in communication that are characteristic of autism. In this way he was more like a child with Asperger's syndrome, but that label didn't fit either because Jeffrey did not have a deficit in reciprocal social interaction. He was not only affectionate toward his parents, as are some young autistic children, but he also tried to act in ways that pleased them. "Mommy, why do I play with strings?" asked this child who would dangle strings in front of his eyes for four hours a day (31). Jeffrey was diagnosed as having obsessive-compulsive disorder, and his stereotyped behavior was controlled with medication.

A father who has guided the care of his severely disabled son for over thirty years said to me, "Yes, my son has autism, but that's just one of his problems." To understand what that father meant we have to consider the concept of comorbidity—co-occurring conditions or behavioral symptoms.

Fragile X syndrome is a disorder defined by a particular genetic marker, namely a fragile site on the X chromosome. This syndrome is associated with mental retardation, and with social and communicative dysfunctions characteristic of autism. The prevalence of fragile X syndrome in the autistic population is higher than would be expected by chance alone.

Walter, the young man whose behavior at a conference reception caught my attention, has fragile X syndrome, a fact that his mother learned only after he was given the simple screening test for this condition that has been available since the early 1990s. As a child, Walter was diagnosed as having autism but no other condition was identified. Today, Walter is considered a man with fragile X syndrome and autism, or fragile X syndrome with autistic characteristics. Little in his life changed because of this revision in his diagnosis after he reached adulthood. He continues to work in a supported employment program operated by an autism center and his relationship to his family remains the same. What does now concern Walter's mother is whether her daughter may be a carrier of fragile X syndrome and could transmit this genetic disorder to any children she may have.

Several other conditions are comorbid with autism, epilepsy among them. These conditions are not found in all individuals with autism, but they do occur at much higher rates than in the general population. From a parent's point of view such comorbidity implies the likelihood of more difficulties and a less optimistic developmental outlook. For the researcher comorbidity is a clue in the search for the causes of autism.

And so, after examining conditions difficult to differentiate from autism, associated with autism, and overlapping with autism we come to the question, what causes autism? As Marie Bristol, a speaker from the National Institutes of Health (NIH) said at a 1996 conference when she addressed this question, "The short answer is that we don't know." But, she added, we have some good hunches. We do know that autism does *not* come from something bad that parents did to their children, but it may come from parents in a different way. One of the strong hunches among researchers today is that autism (or some subcategories of it) is a genetic disorder, or that a susceptibility to autism may be inherited and may be triggered by a variety of factors. Autism also appears to reflect a combination of abnormalities in both structural and functional aspects of the nervous system. Researchers are hard at work trying to identify these abnormalities and locate the genetic factors that may underlie them. We do not yet know the cause or causes of autism, but answers to critical issues surrounding its origins are beginning to emerge.

2 Being Autistic

In 1950 I was labeled autistic and groped my way

from the far side of darkness.

(Grandin and Scariano 1986, 15)

A highly articulate cum laude graduate of one of the most prestigious universities, who was diagnosed as autistic in childhood, had been speaking to his audience for about twenty minutes. "I grew up on the fringes of typical society," he told us. "I always thought I was weird and strange. . . . Many of us wind up on the fringes of society. Even those of us with college degrees are unemployed or underemployed. . . .

"We, whose labels were dropped, are just becoming aware of ourselves," he continued. "There aren't many of us. . . . Some of us have discovered e-mail. We don't have to deal with the anxiety-provoking aspects of conversation—the other person stops and it's your turn. . . . We joke about '1,499 out of every 1,500 people being born with typicality.' . . . When it comes to forming relationships with 'typicals,'" he related, "it doesn't often happen. . . . People sense that something is different."

Individuals with autism are a highly studied population. They are

20

observed and tested, treated and tested; their parents are questioned; their blood is examined, and increasingly so too are their neurological systems, thanks to newer brain-imaging techniques. There are probably thousands of articles on the subject of what goes on inside the minds and bodies of autistic people, and yet the answers are incomplete. We can describe the range of behavioral characteristics of individuals with autism and delineate ways in which their behavior is different, strange, even deficient. We formulate hypotheses to account for these differences and test these hypotheses. Sometimes we even listen to autistic adults as they try to tell us how they have experienced autism.

Autistic individuals describing their experiences? It sounds like a contradiction. Individuals with autism have difficulties in communication, in relating to others; they have little insight or ability to understand others' viewpoints. Are they even aware of how they differ? Autistic people whose ability to communicate is very limited or absent may not help us answer that question, but those individuals who are considered "high-functioning" or "near normal" or "recovered" are aware of these differences, as several have told us in their autobiographical accounts.

Two books and numerous articles and presentations make Temple Grandin the superstar of autistic communicators. In her late forties now, she has come a long way, understanding her differentness and developing strategies to cope with the expectations of the outside world. Donna Williams, with three books, at least one article and several television interviews, is Temple's closest rival, although recently some questions have been raised about Donna's designation as an autistic person (Gollan 1996). Other biographical accounts are more modest—Paul McDonnell's coda to his mother's account of his life; the comments of Sean Barron interwoven with those of his mother in their jointly authored book, and parts of articles or chapters by others.

We are cautioned not to rely too much on the content of these accounts; it may mislead us. We should consider possible limitations in the autistic person's insight, and the applicability of the experiences of this tiny subgroup of highly able autistic individuals (Happe 1991). Yes, it's a skewed sample. It doesn't represent a large segment of the population of autistic individuals; yet we can learn from it. The perspective of these "insiders" may shed light not only on their own experiences but also on those of somewhat less able autistic individuals. Their accounts, used in tandem with the findings of professionals and the perceptions of parents, illuminate the experience of being autistic.

To illustrate the tandem use of insider and outsider perspectives, let's look ıt the thinking of higher functioning individuals with autism or Asperger's syndrome. Temple Grandin, whose most recent book is entitled *Thinking in Pictures*, reports: "Language and words are alien ways of thinking for me. All my thoughts are like playing different tapes in the videocassette recorder in my imagination. Before I researched other people's thinking methods, I assumed that everybody thought in pictures" (1995, 142). Research data and clinical observations support the idea that visual ideation is common among individuals with autism, and many educational programs for young autistic children incorporate visual teaching and learning strategies to capitalize on it. A recent study of introspection in three adults with Asperger's syndrome found that all three described their inner experiences exclusively in visual images, whereas the normal subjects studied earlier had reported multiple types of inner experiences, including verbal thinking. One autistic subject referred to images as the shapes of his thoughts (Hurlburt et al. 1994). Reports of individuals with autism and research by professionals can be used together productively to provide insight into the dynamics of autism.

Certain themes jump out of the biographical accounts of people with autism. They are reiterated over and over by almost every individual. Fear, confusion, and the arduousness of life permeate the descriptions of childhood. Twenty-five years ago an autistic man looking back at his childhood remembered: "Fear was my biggest problem. It was a terrible feeling" (Donovan 1971, 101). Jerry, a thirty-one-year-old man who had been diagnosed as autistic at age four by Leo Kanner, was interviewed about his memories of childhood. He remembered confusion and terror (Bemporad 1979). A twenty-two-year-old man who was diagnosed as autistic at age two writes: "I was afraid of everything!" (Volkmar and Cohen 1985, 49). Donna Williams reports that "the more I became aware of the world around me, the more I became afraid" (1992, 5). Sean Barron writes: "Sometimes I sit and reflect on my life so far. I remember the

fear that was always with me, the confusion, the chaos, and the stormi-
ness of my life with my family" (1992, 257). An eighteen-year-old
woman writes: "In the beginning, when I was a child, life was very
difficult" (DePaolo 1995, 9). A forty-one-year-old man with Asperger's
syndrome reports: "I fear that people are not going to be pleased with
me. I fear that if I do the wrong thing or say the wrong thing I will undo
all the progress I have made so far" (Dewey 1991, 202).

Part of the fear in childhood came from the apparent instability of the
world. Everything appeared to be always changing. "Nothing seemed
constant; everything was unpredictable and strange," reported Jerry
(Bemporad 1979, 192). Paul McDonnell wrote: "When my mom moved
the furniture in the house I got very, very upset. I hated the change. I
felt like I was not at home any more" (1993, 348). Another adult with
autism wrote: "I hate change. I always have, I always will" (McKean
1994, 45).

Rituals are developed to ensure stability and predictability. Everything has to be in a certain place. Events have to occur in a certain order.
People have to act in specified ways. Control becomes critical to ensuring predictability and stability. By setting out exacting prescriptions for
behavior, some individuals with autism have made their homes hellish
for other family members.

Certainty is a goal, but certainty is often evasive. Repetition offers the
key to certainty. Paul McDonnell states:

> In the past I used to ask the same question over and over and I used to
> drive my parents crazy by doing that! I wanted to hear the same answer
> over and over because I was never sure of anything. . . . I wanted an ex-
> act answer to everything; uncertainty used to drive me crazy. (McDon-
> nell 1993, 327)

Sean Barron writes: "I loved repetition. Every time I turned on a light I
knew what would happen. When I flipped the switch, the light went on.
It gave me a wonderful feeling of security because it was exactly the
same each time" (20).

People are not like light switches. They don't act exactly the same
each time. Their behavior cannot be easily understood or predicted by
autistic individuals, particularly not by autistic children. This may be

part of the reason why people may have little meaning for many young children with autism.

> People bothered me. I didn't know what they were for or what they would do to me. They were not always the same and I had no security with them at all. Even a person who was always nice to me might be different sometimes. Things didn't fit together to me with people. Even when I saw them a lot, they were still in pieces, and I couldn't connect them to anything.
>
> Thinking back, I believe that when I was a child, up to the age of five or six, I would not have been able to pick out my mother from a group of other women. I never really looked at her. (Barron and Barron 1992, 20–21)

Negative feelings toward people sometimes developed because people intruded into the special world of the autistic child and interrupted the child's pleasurable and comforting activities. "I hated my mother becaus [sic] she try [sic] to stop me from being in my world and doing what I liked," a young man writes (Volkmar and Cohen 1985, 49). "I remember my mother telling me not to do things I loved," Sean Barron tells us. His parents were always "interrupting me and interfering with me" (21). Donna Williams relates, "I felt secure in 'my world' and hated anything that tried to call me out of there. . . . People, no matter how good, had no chance to compete" (1994b, 8).

What are the experiences that engross and comfort and give pleasure to young autistic children? Donna Williams described her world as the "pleasant, beautiful, and hypnotic experiences of mere color, sensation, and sound" (1992, 129). Temple Grandin gave the following description:

> I could sit on the beach for hours dribbling sand through my fingers. . . . Each particle of sand intrigued me. . . . Other times I scrutinized each line in my finger, following one as if it were a road map.
>
> I enjoyed twirling myself around or spinning coins or lids round and round and round. Intensely preoccupied with the movement of the spinning coin or lid, I saw nothing. . . . People around me were transparent. And no sound intruded on my fixation. (Grandin and Scariano 1986, 22)

Not understanding words or their purpose contributes greatly to the confusion of young children with autism and hinders the development of connectedness to other people. Donna Williams explained this:

> Words were no problem, but other people's expectations for me to respond to them were. This would have required my understanding what was said. . . .
> "What do you think you're doing?" came the voice.
> Knowing I must respond in order to get rid of this annoyance, I would compromise, repeating "What do you think you're doing?" addressed to no one in particular.
> "Don't repeat everything I say," scolded the voice.
> Sensing a need to respond, I'd reply: "Don't repeat everything I say." (Williams 1992, 4)

Bill Donovan, a "near-normal" adult with autism reported, "I learned to talk at 4. I didn't learn to communicate until 11 or 12" (1971, 102). What Bill Donovan meant by this statement was that he, like Donna Williams, parroted words without understanding their meaning or purpose. Not being able to talk was the hardest part of childhood, Bill Donovan relates. "I destroyed things . . . *because I couldn't talk*" (100).

Understanding the speech of others did not guarantee the production of speech. Steffie DePaolo writes: "I am an autistic person and for a long time, I was completely unable to express myself . . . the only solution I had was anger. Then came the tantrums" (1995, 9). "As an autistic child, difficulty in speaking was one of my greatest problems," Temple Grandin relates. "Although I could understand everything people said, my responses were limited. I'd try, but most of the time no spoken words came" (Grandin and Scariano 1986, 18). "My mother and teachers wondered why I screamed. Screaming was the only way I could communicate" (106). Perhaps the worst aspect of not being able to speak, bright autistic children found, was being unable to show how much they knew and understood.

Jim Sinclair, a man completing graduate studies, described his inability to use speech to communicate until he was twelve: "I simply didn't know . . . what talking was for. . . . Speech therapy was just a lot of meaningless drills in repeating meaningless sounds for incomprehensible reasons. I had no idea that this could be a way to exchange meaning with other minds" (1992, 296). Speech, which we think of as an innate ability of human beings, appears to be no more natural to these autistic children than it is for children born deaf.

"Feeling different" is an almost universal experience among those adults who report to us on their feelings. A young man with Asperger's syndrome told one audience that he grew up thinking he had a curse on him. Paul McDonnell writes: "I always knew I was different from other kids, I just didn't know what that difference was. For years I guessed I was retarded, mildly retarded. . . . That's what kids always called me" (327). "I have believed for so long that I was abnormal, retarded, inferior," Sean Barron writes (232). Feelings of "rage, shame, and hatred" toward oneself sometimes accompany this perception (Bovee 1995, 6).

Many individuals with autism who try to explain the ways in which they are different refer to their sensations, to the way they experience sensory input. The common denominator appears to be unusual sensitivity to sensory stimuli and susceptibility to sensory overload—sounds are unbearably loud and sometimes frightening, odors may be overpowering, touch may be painful, sunlight disabling, and combinations of sensory input overwhelming.

The narrative of Darren White begins as follows: "This autobiography consists of information about my hearing and eyesight playing tricks on me" (1987, 224). He then describes these tricks:

> I was rarely able to hear sentences because my hearing distorted them. I was sometimes able to hear a word or two at the start and understand it and then the next lot of words sort of merged into one another and I could not make head or tail of it. . . . Sometimes when other kids spoke to me I could scarcely hear them and sometimes they sounded like bullets. . . .
>
> It was a very bright day and very hot. My eyesight blurred several times that day and once I could see no more than a yard in front. . . . I broke my collarbone falling off a radiator. My eyes were showing a wide windowsill where the radiator was and I sat down falling off instantly. (White and White 1987, 224–25)

A thirteen-year-old boy reports the approach of trains five to ten minutes before they pass his home, long before his parents can hear their approach. This same boy in describing touch reports: "It hurts . . . it's too much" (Cesaroni and Garber 1991, 306).

A mother of an autistic child who herself has characteristics of autism states:

> I have cringed so many times when people came at me for a hug. I taught myself to tolerate this because people always seem to do it. . . . When I am touched unexpectedly or when I do not want to be, I can easily go into overload. This is comparable to having one's chalkboard completely erased and being left to stare at a blank board. At school, if I was touched while I was being taught, my brain immediately shut down. (Donnelly 1994, 7)

Donna Williams as an adult was still frequently overwhelmed by sensory stimulation:

> I had just come from another classroom where I had been tortured by sharp white fluorescent light, which made reflections bounce off everything. It made the room race busily in a constant state of change. Light and shadow dancing on people's faces as they spoke turned the scene into an animated cartoon.
> Now, in this noisy classroom, I felt I was standing at the meeting point of several long tunnels. Blah-blah-blah echoed, bouncing noise wall to wall. I looked at the cheerful, placid faces of the others; clearly I was the freak. (Williams 1994b, 76)

Unusual sensitivity to sensory stimuli is, however, only one of the problems individuals with autism describe. Autism is a pervasive disorder affecting all systems of functioning, Donna Williams reminds us (1994a). To Jim Sinclair the crux of the difference between individuals with autism and others lies in what others know without being taught:

> Simple, basic skills such as recognizing people and things presuppose even simpler, more basic skills such as knowing how to attach meaning to visual stimuli. Understanding speech requires knowing how to process sounds—which first requires recognizing sounds as things that can be processed, and recognizing processing as a way to extract order from

chaos. Producing speech (or producing any other kind of motor behavior) requires keeping track of all the body parts involved, and coordinating all their movements.

Producing any behavior in response to any perception requires monitoring and coordinating all the inputs and outputs at once, and doing it fast enough to keep up with changing inputs that may call for changing outputs. Do you have to remember to plug in your eyes in order to make sense of what you're seeing? . . .

These are the gaps that I notice most often; gaps between what is expected to be learned and what is assumed to be already understood. (1992, 295)

Making sense of emotions is one of these gaps. Paul McDonnell writes, "I just CAN'T understand human emotions, no matter how hard I try" (347). Donna Williams explains:

> I wanted to understand emotions. I had dictionary definitions for most of them and cartoon caricatures of others. . . . I also had trouble reading what other people felt. I could make some translations, though. If people's voices got louder, faster, or went up, they were angry. If tears rolled down their faces, or the sides of their mouths hung down, they were sad. If they were shaking, they were perhaps frightened, sick, or cold. . . .
>
> The most important thing was to check if people were angry. "Angry" had the worst and most invasive consequences. . . . "Are you angry?" I asked Dr. Marek, as his voice changed. "No Donna, I'm not angry," he replied for the fiftieth time. (Williams 1994b, 104)

When Temple Grandin was younger, she could not interpret even the simplest expressions of emotion, Oliver Sacks reports from his meeting with her; she learned to decode such expressions later in her life.

Another of the gaps Jim Sinclair referred to is in making connections. Connections don't come easily to individuals with autism, and this gap affects all aspects of relating to the world. Professionals refer to difficulty with abstraction and generalization. Each event is perceived as distinct from all others. The categorizing that goes on in the minds of most of us all of the time—the automatic connecting of events and people that seem to go together—either doesn't happen or happens in different ways in individuals with autism. Temple Grandin reports that she had to construct her own personal library of these connections, event by event, in order to cope effectively. Donna Williams notes:

> I would learn how to tackle a given situation in one context but be lost when confronted by the same situation in another context. Things just didn't translate. If I learned something while I was standing with a woman in a kitchen and it was summer and it was daytime, the lesson wouldn't be triggered in a similar situation if I was standing with a man in another room and it was winter and it was nighttime. (Williams 1994b, 64).

Difficulty in making connections contributes greatly to one of the core problems in autism, namely reciprocal social interaction. Reciprocal social interaction presupposes a common set of perceptions and understandings that is often missing when autistic and nonautistic adults attempt to communicate. Jim Sinclair reports:

> The extent to which communication occurs in the course of my interactions seems to depend on how effectively I am able to identify discrepancies in understanding and to "translate" both my own and the other person's terms to make sure we're both focusing on the same thing at the same time. (Cesaroni and Garber 1991, 311)

Donna Williams describes her own difficulty in communicating:

> I would often talk on and on about something that interested me. . . . I really was not interested in discussing anything; nor did I expect answers or opinions from the other person, and I would often ignore them or talk over them if they interrupted. . . . If I had to ask questions, it was as though I did so to the air. (Williams 1992, 51)

Communication difficulties and the lack of implicit knowledge of social conventions and codes make the process of connecting with other persons enormously costly in time and energy for the autistic person. Temple Grandin reports that she had to learn these "implicit" social skills, like Data on Star Trek.

> I am like Data, the android man, on "Star Trek, the Next Generation." As he accumulates more information, he has a greater understanding of

social relationships. I am a scientist who has to learn the strange ways of an alien culture. . . . When I encounter a new social situation, I have to scan my memory and look for previous experiences that were similar. As I accumulate more memories, I become more and more skilled at predicting how other people will act in a particular situation. (Grandin 1995, 147)

It is the absence of this common set of perceptions and understandings, the implicit knowledge of social conventions and codes acquired during the course of childhood and adolescent development in most individuals, that leads to reports by autistic individuals of feeling alien. Temple Grandin, who supplied the title for the Oliver Sacks book *An Anthropologist on Mars* in the course of describing her experiences, was not the first and far from the only adult with autism to use an alien metaphor in trying to describe the autistic experience. Jim Sinclair reports:

After reading Temple Grandin's autobiography . . . someone asked me if I thought a cattle chute would have helped me. I said I didn't need a cattle chute, I needed an orientation manual for extraterrestrials. Being autistic does not mean being inhuman. But it does mean being alien. It means that what is normal for other people is not normal for me, and what is normal for me is not normal for other people. In some ways I am terribly ill-equipped to survive in this world, like an extraterrestrial stranded without an orientation manual. (1992, 302)

Sean Barron tells us that at age fifteen, "I still didn't have a clue as to how people talked to one another. Not for the first time, I felt like an alien from outer space—I had no more idea how to communicate with people than a creature from another planet" (198).

In somewhat less striking language, other adults communicate similar experiences of not being able to understand the commonplace codes of human behavior. A woman with a graduate degree reports: "I was never *quite* sure how to handle certain situations. It is very difficult for even a high-functioning autistic adult to know exactly when to say something, when to ask for help, or when to remain quiet. To such a person, life is a game in which the rules are constantly changing without rhyme or reason" (Carpenter 1992, 291).

Yet at some point all these individuals decided to try to "make it" in the alien world of "typicals," to find some way to learn the rules and develop the necessary skills and coping mechanisms. For some, this happened at a clear point in time as a clear, conscious decision. Imitation of typical people was a major strategy to accomplish their goal.

> I was 14. I set my will (to) be normal like everybody else. (I) look(ed) up to people in school and did what they did to be accepted and put (up) more of a show to hide the problems and be Normal. . . . My interests were destroyed becouse [sic] I thought they wernt [sic] normal. (Volkmar and Cohen 1985, 51)

Sean Barron writes:

> I spent an awful lot of time wishing I were a different person. Why couldn't I be normal? More than anything I wanted to change all my behavior. . . . I started having "corrective" conversations with myself.
>
> I went on a crusade. . . . I declared war! I was going to fight against all the behaviors I had obeyed all my life. (Barron and Barron 1992, 161, 232)

Some autistic persons have more ambivalence about trying to be normal. In an author's note at the beginning of her book *Nobody Nowhere*, Donna Williams writes:

> This is a story of two battles, a battle to keep out of "the world" and a battle to join it. It tells of the battles within my own world and the battle lines, tactics used, and the casualties of my private war against others.
>
> This is my attempt at a truce, the conditions of which are on my terms. (Williams 1992)

She had learned, Donna Williams wrote, that her survival rested on "refining the act of acting normal"; but "on the inside I knew that by definition this meant that whatever and whoever I was naturally was unworthy of acceptance, belonging, or even life" (1992, 80). In a television interview on CBS in 1994 Donna Williams talked about giving up the mimicry of others that was central to her attempt to learn to live in the normal world so that she could find her own self; she is no longer willing to maintain a facade of normality.

"Being almost 'normal' is not easy," Jean-Paul Bovee tells us (1995, 6). Jim Sinclair tells us more about this, his dreams and his disappointments, in his poem:

> I built a bridge
> out of nowhere, across nothingness
> and wondered if there would be something on the other side.
> I built a bridge
> out of fog, across darkness
> and hoped that there would be light on the other side.
> I built a bridge
> out of despair, across oblivion
> and knew that there would be hope on the other side.
> I built a bridge out of helplessness, across chaos
> and trusted that there would be strength on the other side.
> I built a bridge
> out of hell, across terror
> and it was a good bridge, a strong bridge,
> a beautiful bridge.
> It was a bridge I built myself,
> with only my hands for tools, my obstinacy for supports
> my faith for spans, and my blood for rivets.
> I built a bridge, and crossed it,
> but there was no one there to meet me on the other side.
>
> (Cesaroni and Garber 1991, 311–12)

Thomas McKean puts it another way in his poem "Build Me a Bridge": he comes from a different world; he wants to be part of this world; but he, himself, can't build the bridge needed to join that world.

> I have known that you and I
> have never been quite the same.
> And I used to look up at the stars at night
> and wonder which one was from where I came.
> Because you seem to be part of another world
> and I will never know what it's made of.
> Unless you build me a bridge, build me a bridge,
> build me a bridge out of love. . . .
>
> (McKean 1994, 43)

♂ Life Cycles

What can I expect for my child's future? parents ask—or fear to ask but are told anyhow. Frequently, the forecast includes continued significant impairment, multiple problems, separateness from nondisabled peers, and lifelong special service needs. This picture is sometimes what the future holds for autistic children, but not always; and a bleak future looms before autistic children much less often today than ten or twenty years ago. No single pattern of development and adult outcome characterizes the autistic condition. There are many possible patterns, and many factors—some controllable, some not—shape the patterns. Parents need to know this fact. So too do the physicians and others—professionals and nonprofessionals—who interact with autistic children and their families. This chapter addresses some of the developmental patterns noted in autistic individuals.

INFANTS AND TODDLERS

Until recently, when the urgent need for early intervention was recognized, the diagnosis of autism was usually deferred until a child was three years of age. No speech at age two: "Give your child a chance," doctors would say; "children develop at different rates." No reaching out to others: "Some children are shy; you're being overanxious." By two-and-a-half years they might add, "He's a little slow developmentally." But the mothers of these children often knew, or at least strongly suspected, that something was seriously wrong, and in many cases they sensed this almost from the time they brought their babies home. How did they know? What were the clues they "picked up" that others did not recognize until much later?

Differences in babies' temperaments are apparent even in their first days of life. Some infants are quite fussy, while others lie quietly, hardly moving; some cry most of the time as if in great discomfort, while others cry only occasionally and with less vigor; some can be soothed easily by being picked up or fed, while others seem impervious to almost all attempts to soothe them. Researchers have studied these differences in characteristic behavior and have found them to reflect long-lasting patterns of behavior.

No single pattern of infant behavior characterizes babies who were later identified as autistic. But two patterns are commonly reported: the very easy or "perfect" baby—quiet, undemanding, apparently content with little attention from caregivers—and the very irritable baby who resists soothing and does not establish eye contact. Some of these babies don't like being held and reject all attempts at cuddling or other forms of physical contact, even arching their bodies away from their parents. Of course, many babies with these early patterns grow into happy and healthy children; there is no one-to-one correspondence between these early patterns and later outcomes. Just the same, these early patterns provide a kind of first alert that a baby may need some special help with its development.

Tony was an irritable baby who was later recognized as having autistic characteristics. In her book, *Fighting for Tony,* Mary Callahan described the constant crying that marked his first two-and-a-half years.

> Each day Tony's crying spells grew longer and more frequent. . . . Most days he cried for an hour or two in the morning, about four at dinnertime and another hour during the night. . . . Our pediatrician talked of colic and immature nervous systems. He said it wouldn't last more than six weeks. On the day that Tony turned six weeks old, I took him to the doctor in the middle of what turned out to be nine straight hours of crying. (Callahan 1987, 20, 21)

Let's look at some of the other early clues that infants with autism may provide. Right from the start, something very basic about relating to people seems not to be working. Typical characteristics of children diagnosed as autistic under age three include little or no eye contact; lack of responsiveness to speech (often leading to suspicion of deafness); and apparent obliviousness to people.

The normally developing infant turns toward an adult who begins speaking and studies that person's face. The baby smiles at and vocalizes to its mother. After a while the infant adds anticipatory gestures, lifting its arms to be picked up. A pattern of reciprocal interaction develops, with mother and baby being the focus of each other's attention and regulating their behavior in response to each other. When the baby cries, the mother is soothing. When the mother is playful, the baby smiles or laughs.

The parent's face becomes a source of important information for the baby in situations of uncertainty, as when a new toy is presented or an unfamiliar adult seeks close contact. This process of social referencing, that is, getting cues from the parent or other caregiver, helps guide the infant's responses. Near the end of the first year the infant also intentionally uses communicative signals to direct the parent's attention to interesting objects and events, to share those experiences. The infant may point to a dog passing by or hold out a toy and vocalize, then check to find out if the adult is looking at it. This joint attention, along with social referencing and reciprocal interaction, provides the foundation for later social relatedness and communication.

Infants with autism rarely if ever take part in this joint attention, social referencing, and reciprocal interactive behavior between mother and baby. In the case of late-onset autism, such behaviors are lost or significantly reduced sometime after the first year. Autistic babies don't effectively use eye contact, facial expressions, and gestures in relating to their parents and others as do normally developing infants. Nor does the human voice appear to carry special meaning or attract any special attention. One theory to explain this difference is that the process of regulating arousal is impaired in the autistic infant, and one of the staunchest supporters of this theory is Stanley Greenspan.

Stanley Greenspan, M.D., child psychiatrist and faculty member of the George Washington University School of Medicine, is considered by many to be the mentor of developmental intervention with very young children. Based on his work with hundreds of infants and toddlers, Greenspan developed two concepts that are relevant to the understanding of pervasive developmental disorders, namely "regulatory disorder" and "multisystem developmental disorder" (Greenspan 1992b; Zero to Three 1994).

A regulatory disorder is an inability to process sensations, that is, to take them in, modulate (adapt to) them, and comprehend them, while staying calm and attentive. Infants with regulatory disorders may over- or underreact to noises and bright lights; may show "tactile defensiveness," stiffening and arching their bodies to avoid the physical handling involved in being dressed or held; may under- or overreact to pain; and often have severe difficulty with auditory processing and the processing of multisensory experiences. With different kinds of words Greenspan describes the early sensory experiences reported by Donna Williams, Temple Grandin, Sean Barron, Paul McDonnell, Jim Sinclair, and other persons with autism we encountered in the previous chapter.

Greenspan believes that severe regulatory dysfunction interferes with communication and the formation of relationships by hindering the development of shared attention and reciprocal gesturing between a baby and his or her parents. Thus, his concept of a "multisystem developmental disorder," which involves problems in language, social relationships, and motor planning, links these problems to sensory processing difficulties.

Why does this connection matter? What implication does it have? Let's consider the finding that many infants with autism appear to show little interest in the human face, or that autistic children may not recognize their parents until well beyond the age when most normally developing babies can, even well beyond the point when most mentally retarded babies can differentiate their parents from strangers. Greenspan's explanation might point out that the visual image of the human face usually appears to an infant simultaneously with auditory, tactile, and often kinesthetic stimuli; parents talk or sing to their babies while they stroke or rock them and seek to establish eye contact. Thus, the infant who can't cope with multisensory stimuli may be overwhelmed and react by "turning off" human faces.

Greenspan's conceptualization has implications for the selection of early intervention strategies. For example, an initial intervention strategy would be to carefully observe the baby's responses to various stimuli, and to reduce the types and levels of stimulation that appear to upset the infant or cause him to withdraw, while providing the sensory stimulation he seems to favor. Later, the baby would be very gradually reintroduced to the types of stimuli he didn't tolerate well.

Geraldine Dawson of the University of Washington also believes that the baby's ability to adapt to various types, levels, and combinations of sensory stimuli is central to its healthy development (1991). Normally developing infants react to people and other stimuli with orienting or with aversive responses—turning toward and attending to the stimulus, or turning away from a person or object. An orienting response is the typical reaction to stimuli of mild intensity like soft speech and gentle rocking, while the aversive response is a common response to very intense stimuli like loud shouting. Autistic infants may, however, have abnormal arousal patterns: stimuli that arouse interest in most babies may meet an aversive response such as gaze avoidance in the autistic baby.

Is the optimal level of novelty lower for the autistic infant? Most infants are interested in stimuli that are slightly different from what they have previously experienced but not ones that are totally novel. What they seem to seek are a few familiar features. Thus, we could conceive of an optimal level of novelty along with an optimal range of stimulation. For autistic children, the optimal level of novelty may be lower. This possibility is supported by both the marked distress that autistic children show over minor changes in their environments and by their restricted range of interests. The narrow range of optimal stimulation and novelty for autistic children may also help explain their difficulty in understanding people and participating in social situations. Novelty and unpredictability are much more closely associated with social stimuli than with objects.

As the autistic child moves from infancy/toddlerhood to the preschool years, ages three to five, we see a child who lacks a foundation for social interaction and communication, and who may well have problems in modulating stimuli. Some new areas of delayed or deviant development are also likely to become apparent: the absence of age-appropriate play and the presence of stereotyped behaviors, that is, repetitive motor sequences that have no obvious function, like hand flapping. They mark an inauspicious entry to the preschool years.

THE PRESCHOOL YEARS

> There is no question that the evolution of spoken language as we know it was a defining point in human prehistory. Perhaps it was *the* defining point. Equipped with language, humans were able to create new kinds of worlds in nature: The world of introspective consciousness and the world we manufacture and share with others, which we call "culture."
>
> *(Leakey 1994, 119)*

By three years of age most children have joined this world we share with others, and their most powerful medium for sharing is speech. Normally developing three-year-olds use speech for a variety of purposes such as making their needs known, gathering information, sharing information, and directing and controlling others. An autistic child, lacking an organized system of communication, cannot partake of this shared world.

By the time a child approaches three years of age and still lacks meaningful speech, family practitioners and pediatricians as well as parents have usually agreed on the need for a diagnostic evaluation by a specialist in childhood disorders. With federal education law mandating the provision of special education services to preschoolers with disabilities, and with early intervention services to infants and toddlers with developmental delays also available, many three-year-olds have already been diagnosed and are already receiving special education services. The characteristic that most often drives this process is the child's lack of meaningful or functional speech. Furthermore, a critical precursor of speech, namely communicative intent, may be absent.

Communicative intent, the motivation to communicate with others, does not, in itself, assure the development of speech or language. Some children with profound mental retardation display communicative intent but acquire only a few words or manual signs. However, communicative intent is the sine qua non for functional speech. What complicates this situation is the difficulty in differentiating a lack of communicative intent from a severe impairment in the ability to process language, understand its function and meaning, and organize a communicative act, whether through speech, gesture, or sign.

A lack of communicative intent is sometimes used as the central explanation for the absence of speech and gestures in a preschool child with autism. The reminiscences of some adults with autism, Donna Williams and Sean Barron, for example, who report that they much preferred their own worlds to the outside world, seem to support this idea. However, other adults cited in chapter 2 report very different experiences. Bill Donovan and Steffie DePaolo vividly remembered their inability to produce speech in early childhood in spite of intense efforts to do so. Some young autistic children do speak, but only on rare occasions. This too is often attributed to weak motivation to communicate to others, but Temple Grandin and other adults with autism report that their intervals without speech resulted largely from continuing, sporadic difficulty in producing speech.

The production of speech is a motor as well as a cognitive act. Even the use of gestures or signs requires the child to organize what he or she wants to communicate and to coordinate the appropriate motor actions. Difficulties can arise at any stage of this process, and children with disabilities other than autism also sometimes display motor-planning problems.

A situation I observed almost thirty years ago illustrates this point. A boy of six or seven was being evaluated at a pediatric language disorder clinic. One part of this examination was a diagnostic teaching task in which the child was taught to recognize three written words and was then asked to pick them out from a small pack of word cards presented one by one. The specific directions given by the examiner were, "Stop me when you see one of these words." Twice the examiner went slowly through the pack of word cards without being stopped. Her conclusion was that the child had not learned the three words well enough to remember them and distinguish them from the other words. He had failed the task.

At that point the director of the clinic, who had been observing the evaluation, asked to take over. She gave the boy a wooden mallet from a toy workbench and instructed him, "Bang on this table hard when you see one of the words." This time the boy banged his mallet three times, once in response to each of the words he had been taught. What had been interpreted by the first examiner to be a learning problem now appeared to be a problem in coordinating and implementing a response.

To varying degrees motivation, cognition, and motor-planning abilities may all affect the delayed or deviant speech of individual children with autism. Slowness in organizing a response appears to be an issue that goes beyond the establishment of speech. This difficulty has been noted in verbal children with autism and in some high-functioning adults. Over fifty years ago Leo Kanner, who introduced the concept of autism, referred to a bright six-year-old boy with autism whose characteristic response to being asked to describe his experiences was, "Wait, I have to get it in my mind first" (1973, 91).

Language has many functions. A young child can use language to ask for attention, help, or affection; to request food or toys; to share interesting events; to protest. Both the very young child and the child who has not yet acquired a language system such as speech, sign language, or a picture communication system use prelanguage means to achieve these goals. The autistic preschooler without language may vocalize, grab, or manipulate another person's hand as if it were a tool to get food or toys. Tantrums, physical attacks, or self-injury may take the place of speech in protesting movement from favored to disliked activities or in response to any kind of sudden change. Such prelanguage means of communication are often not only inefficient in bringing about the child's objective but also create negative emotional associations between child and caregiver. They sometimes work all too well, establishing maladaptive behavior patterns that further damage the child and limit his potential independence in home, school, and the larger community. For these reasons, parents and professionals should make an intensive effort to facilitate the child's language—both for understanding the communications of others and for expressing himself to others—during the preschool years.

Echolalia, or the echoing of speech, is common in autistic children who have no significant problems with the motor aspects of speech production but have difficulty understanding and using the units of speech in a meaningful way. Richard was a six-year-old with autism at a residential school who loved his psychiatrist. On Monday mornings Dr. S. came to the classroom where I taught, to take Richard for his weekly "therapy" session. Referring to the boy's weekend at his family home, he frequently asked, "Where have you been, Richard?" After a while when Dr. S. appeared at my classroom door Richard would say, "Where you da been Richard?" This was his reproduction of Dr. S.'s way of greeting him, and it appeared to serve both affective and communicative functions, something like "Hi, Dr. S. I'm so glad to see you again. Now let's go for our session together." Then Richard would take Dr. S.'s hand and lead him out of the classroom.

Kevin was a classmate of Richard's, but he did have some functional speech. He made requests, was beginning to attempt simple questions, and used an emphatic "No" to decline some requests from others. Kevin also loved watching television and would periodically repeat jingles, program introductions, and closing remarks from television commercials and shows. These echolalic episodes seemed to give him pleasure while his functional speech continued to emerge and expand.

Echolalia may serve a variety of purposes for young children. It may represent a primitive attempt to communicate for children who have not been able to grasp how meaning is conveyed through language. Echolalic children may be learning language by memorizing and repeating multiword chunks, initially with only general associations to situations or actions. Many of these children will eventually break down the chunks into smaller units and use them more appropriately. In addition, there is evidence that echolalia is more likely to occur in certain situations, for example, when the child is in an unfamiliar situation. Thus, echolalia in a young child with little or no functional speech should not be viewed as pathological behavior that needs to be stamped out. Instead, it should be viewed as a reflection of a point in language development, with recognition given to the functions it may serve. Sometimes this developmental path is clearly visible, as it was with Kenneth, the echolalic five-year-old referred to at the beginning of chapter 1. When Kenneth began to develop functional speech his interactions often went like this:

Mother: "Do you want milk?"

Kenneth: "Do you want milk? Yes."

After a while Kenneth was able to answer "yes" without first echoing his mother's question.

Not all autistic children develop echolalia. Some remain mute or acquire only a handful of word approximations. In the past about 50 percent of individuals with autism failed to develop meaningful speech. With the emphasis on early identification and intervention that has occurred since the late 1980s, and the intensification of educational services to infants, toddlers, and preschoolers with autism or other pervasive developmental disorders that has characterized the mid-to-late 1990s, this percentage has begun to decline significantly.

When a young child with autism responds appropriately to a spoken request, the child may be using cues other than words to guide his responses. This occurs most often in the context of common routines, where speech may serve primarily as an alerting signal. Thus, the child may respond appropriately to his mother's request that he "Come here now; it's time to work" even though he doesn't understand her words. What may be guiding his response is the routine of his mother being seated at a particular table with his chair facing hers, a situation that occurs several times each afternoon. Understanding speech involves breaking the stream of speech sounds into discrete units in accordance with the rules of a particular language. To autistic children who haven't cracked the language code, speech may be a continuous flow of sounds, an undifferentiated chunk of stimuli punctuated by periods of silence.

When communications are too complex for the young autistic child to understand, even with the assistance of situational cues, the child may well tune out the speech directed at him. Sometimes this tuning out by the child is interpreted by the adult as refusal by the child to follow the adult's directions. This situation can escalate into a destructive interaction between the child and caregiver, with the adult becoming insistent and angry and the child becoming anxious and perhaps engaging in aggressive or self-injurious behavior. If such interactions are to be minimized, parents, teachers, and others must understand the child's level of language comprehension and use language well within that range. The exception to this general rule is carefully planned instruction targeted at expanding language skills, which pushes at the boundaries of the child's current level of language comprehension.

While young autistic children have severe difficulty with most aspects of language, a small number of autistic preschoolers learn to read or at least to recite words correctly from the written page, often with little or no formal instruction, to the amazement of their parents and teachers. A three-year-old with no speech, who made few attempts at communicating with others, was observed using plastic letters to form words that he had previously seen on the television screen. At age four, after he had learned to name some objects, this boy would identify the words he had constructed with his letters. Visual-spatial skills and visual memory are areas of strength in many autistic children. Hyperlexia, or early reading not expected on the basis of IQ or language development, reflects these strengths.

Hyperlexia is a term that carries some negative connotations. In the past some professionals denigrated this ability in various ways, perceiving it as a rote skill that had no functional value. That view has changed as professionals recognized that such early, unexpected reading was often more than just word naming; and that even when the child's comprehension of the words he was reading was poor, this skill may be beneficial. Freed from the need to teach word recognition, teachers can concentrate on developing better comprehension in these children. In fact, hyperlexia appears to be associated with better developmental outcomes. Moreover, early reading provides the young autistic child with a skill easily recognized by typical peers, a situation that can work to the child's advantage when he or she is included in such mainstream settings as preschool, kindergarten, or first grade.

While some autistic infants and toddlers appear to look through people, treat them as tools, and not recognize their parents, by age three or four most autistic children have begun to relate to selected others—parents, siblings, and perhaps a grandparent. Clara Park describes this change in her daughter Jessy. At age two Jessy appeared for the most part to look at her parents and siblings "as through a pane of glass." By the time she was three her "flashes of response" had become more frequent, and her indifference to her mother had turned into "a kind of attachment," with Jessy following her mother from room to room (1986, 83–84). What remains distinctive about the behavior of preschool children with autism, even when compared to mentally retarded children, is their lack of interest in other children and their odd, impoverished play.

Normally developing toddlers who are brought together are likely to make social overtures to one another. They may smile, offer a toy, or take a toy. While playing separately they may have occasional brief interactions. By age four their play changes markedly, with cooperative play common and make-believe play dominating their joint endeavors. Preschoolers engage in pretend play themes of cooking and eating, doing housework and shopping, being firefighters or bus drivers or doctors, and being sick. At the same age, children with autism are likely to ignore peers, and their version of play is likely to be repetitive, inflexible manipulation of objects and object parts—lining them up, spinning them, or diddling with them.

A variety of explanations have been suggested to account for autistic children's distinctive play pattern. Given the fact that many young autistic children have little or no language and develop slowly in other areas as well, we might attribute play differences to these developmental delays. However, even studies in which autistic children have been compared to other children with similar mental ages or language abilities find these distinctions in play patterns. Several researchers offer another explanation, namely that autistic children have difficulty in overriding the reality-based features of their environment and shifting to internal representations not closely tied to these features, a process basic to make-believe play. In pretend play a doll is a baby, and that baby is fed with a bottle that contains no milk; a child has a conversation with someone on a toy telephone when no one is on the other end; the child goes to "sleep" while actually awake and not in bed. Pretend play has an "as if" quality. It veers from the here-and-now reality of the child's situation. Most preschool children can make this shift easily and enjoy doing so. Young autistic children appear to have difficulty with this process of engaging in play schemes not tied to their immediate situations.

Another factor may also be relevant here. The play of young children is based to a large extent on imitation of actions performed by others, either in past situations or in the present. Imitation, which is a fundamental mode of learning, appears to be an ability that some children with autism don't develop naturally. They have to be taught this skill, which normally developing infants exhibit.

Before turning to the middle years of childhood let's meet a young boy, Ned Christopher, whose early years seemed very promising, and then check back on Tony Callahan, whose early years had seemed less so. Many TV viewers knew Ned's father, William Christopher, as Father Mulcahy of *M*A*S*H*. What these viewers did not know was that his (adopted) son Ned was diagnosed at age three as having atypical development with autistic features. Yet to his parents and some professionals Ned's disability seemed very mild in spite of some unusual behavior.

> "Did you ever hear of a kid who didn't like piggyback?" said his frustrated father. No, he didn't like piggyback, just as he hadn't liked being cuddled when he was a tiny infant. He hadn't liked it, and he had stiffened his little body into a board, making it impossible to cuddle him. (Christopher and Christopher 1989, 12)

But before age three Ned could write the letters of the alphabet, was trying to dress himself independently, and demanded to be told the name of every flag he saw by shouting "flag." He rocked in bed as he slept, but he could recognize and name vegetables and plants in the yard and neighborhood. He didn't respond to strangers who said "Hi" or asked what his name was, but he could count to forty. By age three he could spell and read about fifty words, but he had begun to pull the hair of the little girls in his nursery school class, which was the only time he interacted with any of his classmates. A regular kindergarten class was the goal at that point. In the meantime Ned spent mornings in a special education program with a behavioral approach and continued afternoons in a nursery school. By the end of that year a regular kindergarten program no longer appeared to be a possibility. Shortly before Ned turned six his mother wrote: "Even though his language, behavior, abilities all move forward, it just isn't coming together. . . . Perhaps it is that as he grows older, the gap between Ned and a normal child becomes more obvious" (69).

Tony's progress through the preschool years was quite different. By age four, prodded and instructed by his younger sister, Renee, Tony had begun to engage in dramatic play and conversation. Renee and Tony are playing at giving "juice" to a doll when the following conversation occurs:

RENEE: I spill it.
TONY: No spilling it.
RENEE: I have to.
TONY: You don't have to.
RENEE: Yea, I have to.

TONY: No, you don't have to.

RENEE: Yea.

TONY: No, you don't have to.

RENEE: I have to (screaming).

TONY: I be mad at you. (Callahan 1987, 118)

At age five, with more than a year in a special preschool program, Tony was still not talking to his classmates; he didn't understand them, he told his mother. After months of work on auditory processing with his mother, Tony entered a regular kindergarten class; the school staff knew nothing about his earlier diagnosis of autism. Six weeks later his anxious mother, afraid of what she would learn the following day at a parent-teacher conference, asked the teacher aide how Tony was doing. "'Tony?' she responded with a puzzled look. 'He's doing great. I wish we had a classroom full of kids like Tony. Why?'" (164).

MIDDLE CHILDHOOD

Nellie was again biting her already callused hand. She made noises that sounded like anger. I was new to working with children like Nellie, having previously taught kindergarten and first grade in a public school. I tried to protect Nellie from herself, to take her hand from her mouth. When I finally succeeded, her jaws closed forcefully on my thumb. I struggled to extract it. Her resistance and power astonished me. Nellie was a small girl of six-and-a-half but I feared that I would not see that thumb in one piece again. After a couple of minutes Nellie relaxed her jaw slightly, and I managed to extract my thumb, damaged but still whole.

For most children the middle childhood years are a time of expansion, of moving into the world of formal education and the world of peers; a time for hard work and close friendships. For some autistic children too the years from five or six to about twelve are a period of learning and expansion, but during the early part of this time span diverging paths become apparent, one pointing toward the possibility of near-normal functioning (or perhaps even recovery), the other with an unclear endpoint but with a much greater likelihood of continued significant disability.

Nellie seemed to be on this second path. She rarely spoke and then only in single words or short phrases that voiced demands, usually for food. During Nellie's preschool years her limited and infrequent communication had not seemed to be as serious a problem as it did now, and her hands had not yet become callused from being bitten. At age six these behaviors began to seem much more abnormal. Taken together with the limited progress she had made during the previous year, they damaged her family's hopes for her future as well as the optimism of the professional team responsible for Nellie's treatment.

Self-abusive behavior is not uncommon in individuals with autism, although it is not characteristic of most autistic children or adults. During the middle childhood years both self-injurious behavior and aggression toward others may become more apparent and more difficult to cope with or control. Head-banging has been noted in normally developing infants and toddlers, as well as in babies who are later diagnosed as autistic. In normally developing young children, this behavior occurs mostly at bedtime and disappears altogether before age three, whereas in some autistic children head-banging may occur at various times of the day during varied activities and may increase as the child gets older. A variety of reasons have been proposed to explain this behavior, including the attention and concern it gains the child, the escape from disliked activities it achieves, and the sensory stimulation it provides. Head-banging, or other types of self-injurious behavior, sometimes accompanies medical problems such as frequent severe earaches, which the autistic child with little functional language has no way of reporting. Neurochemical disturbances, particularly dysfunctions in neurotransmitter systems, have also been hypothesized as causing or contributing to self-injurious behavior; and research on stereotyped behavior has pointed to a connection between such behavior and self injury under some conditions that appear to involve the neurotransmitter serotonin (Lewis et al. 1996). Frontal lobe seizures are another hypothesized cause of self-injurious behavior in some individuals with autism, although there is no hard evidence to back up this theory.

When six-year-old Sean was placed in my class, his forehead was bumpy and bruised. During the first few weeks I feared for his vision because he banged his head against the glass windows many times, and I anticipated that one day the glass would break from the force of those blows. I don't know what motivated this self-abuse: perhaps fear, perhaps his inability to communicate his needs, perhaps in part the concern his behavior generated. Whatever the cause, his head-banging declined dramatically after a while as other behaviors emerged. Sean and I played interactive infant games like variants of peek-a-boo, and he giggled when my face reappeared. He imitated my block stacking, and we both laughed when the stacks fell down. Sean began calling me something that resembled "ma ma" when he wanted my attention. Still, one day when he entered the classroom and tripped on his untied shoelace Sean began to bang his head against the floor.

Self-injurious behavior can become entrenched and difficult to eliminate. Yet with skilled intervention self-injury can be significantly reduced in virtually all autistic children. In the last fifteen years or so a whole system of functional analysis has evolved for identifying the factors that may precipitate or maintain self-injurious behavior and for designing treatment strategies to eliminate them. Medication may need to be part of the treatment package in selected cases, although it should be noted that medication may sometimes trigger or increase self-injurious behavior.

> The autistic child presents a singular puzzle: a human being whose conversational language and social skills generally lag way behind apparent intellectual ability. Everywhere else one looks in the human domain, even among those with low IQ, social contact and conversational fluency seem to develop so effortlessly that it looks as if they required no particular skill at all. (Bruner and Feldman 1993, 273)

A major shift in mental functioning occurs between ages five and seven or eight in most children. By the end of this period language has become their vehicle of thought, and their thinking has become more logical. At this time too children become much more skilled at recognizing the codes of social behavior and acting in accordance with them.

Children with autism (or Asperger's syndrome) who have acquired functional language before seven or eight can apply their energies to academic achievement and to learning the rules of social behavior. Autistic children who have not learned to understand speech and to express themselves through speech or another language system are likely to make slow progress in almost all areas of development.

In the middle childhood years the wide diversity within the autistic population becomes strikingly apparent. While some autistic children are still nonverbal, others have acquired large vocabularies; while some still appear unable to understand speech that would make sense to most toddlers, others appear to have close to age-appropriate language comprehension. Some autistic children learn to read as preschoolers, perhaps with only limited comprehension of what they are reading; others may understand written language, as shown by their ability to answer questions based on the written text, even though they do not speak. Irrespective of their differences in acquiring language, one area of communication in which most children with autism show poor skills is conversation. They may be able to talk, but they can't converse.

Conducting a conversation is something most children learn to do with little formal instruction. Parents and teachers of preschoolers may have to say "Wait your turn" or "Give someone else a turn" from time to time, and occasionally an adult may be heard coaching a child with "Why don't you ask _____ about what he watched on television yesterday?" But these kinds of casual reminders in natural situations are all the instruction most young children need. Yet autistic youngsters may need instruction in a range of skills involved in conducting conversations, including how to identify a suitable topic, start a conversation, establish eye contact, attend to what the other person is saying, respond to what the other person is saying, take turns, use appropriate gestures, facial expressions, and proximity, and end a conversation.

Friendships become very important in the middle childhood years, but most autistic children don't form close relationships with peers during this period. One of the reasons why this may be so is that autistic children may lack or be slow in developing a faculty referred to as "theory of mind." What this term signifies is a capacity to understand mental states, for example, beliefs, intentions, feelings, hopes, pretense, and to interpret behavior in terms of mental states. Since this ability appears in all normally developing children without explicit teaching, it is considered an innate capacity or mechanism governed by a particular part of the brain. The absence of this ability to understand what people know, think, and feel may be at the root of some of the difficulties that autistic individuals have in communication and relationships across the life span. We can make sense of the behavior of others because we can think about their thinking, and therefore anticipate their responses to various situations and interactions. Richard Leakey identifies this ability to predict the behavior of others as the central challenge for individuals in primate society. To an autistic child who cannot take into consideration how others are likely to feel, think, or react, the social world must be a perplexing and terrifying place in which to exist—a message that several adults with autism communicated to us in chapter 2.

During middle childhood many autistic children start seeking out other children. One mother reported the following episode after her high-functioning autistic son had invited another boy to his home to play:

> There they were outside on the swing set and the next time I looked up, he was in his room lining up figures, and the friend was just left sitting on the swing set. He had no idea that it wasn't cool to do that, even though we talked about it 100 times. (Church and Coplan 1995, 27)

This behavior reflects the tenuous connection of autistic children to peers and illustrates the theory of mind deficit that may underlie it, at least to some degree. A theory of mind deficit may also be responsible for the naïveté observed in many autistic children, which often reflects an inability to read intentions, as is illustrated by the following example:

> Samantha, a ten-year-old girl with autism attending a mainstream school, was deliberately teased by the children there, and frequently they would tell her to perform some unacceptable act, such as taking her clothes off in the playground. She was quite bewildered by the laughter that ensued . . . believing that her compliance would result in them becoming "her friend." (Baron-Cohen and Howlin 1993, 467)

Similarly, the long monologues of some older autistic children as well as adolescents and adults that cause the persons they are addressing to seek escape may reflect an inability to sense their listeners' level of interest; and the embarrassment or hurt inflicted on others by autistic individuals may reflect an inability to anticipate how their comments will affect other people.

> One young man . . . complained that he couldn't "mind-read." He went on to explain that other people seemed to have a special sense by which they could read other people's thoughts and could anticipate their responses and feelings; he knew this because they managed to avoid upsetting people whereas he was always putting his foot in it, not realizing that he was doing or saying the wrong thing until after the other person became angry or upset. (Rutter 1983, 526)

What is accomplished by giving a name—theory of mind—to a capacity that appears to be absent or underdeveloped in many autistic individuals? The processes of prevention, cure, and treatment are all shaped by understanding; and understanding of core or primary characteristics of autism may both lead to improved treatment and illuminate the search for the neurobiological factors underlying this condition. Is a theory of mind deficit a core characteristic of autism? For more than a decade researchers have explored this question. The best current data indicate that somewhere between 40 and 80 percent of autistic children can't predict the beliefs of others on the same tests passed by normally developing and mentally retarded children of similar mental ages. Thus, at the present time the construct of a theory of mind deficit in autism appears to be a useful way of looking at and studying some of the difficulties in interactive communication and social relationships experienced by children and adults with autism. A few years from now, after we learn more about autism, we may identify a more productive way of viewing these difficulties and other ones.

Middle childhood is also the period when the special abilities of some autistic children become very apparent. A parent described the skill her son had developed at age five in opening locks:

When our son was about five, he had exceptional skill with locks. . . . One day we took him to the grocery store that happened to have a large safe. It immediately drew his attention. I told my son to get away from the lock. However, the clerk intervened to say that it was okay for him to play with it because it was an expensive burglar-proof safe that he couldn't damage. . . .

I think I made it through the first aisle before the alarms went off as the huge safe door began to swing open. Both the clerk and the store manager stood there with their mouths open. (Gilpin 1994, 30–31)

By the age of six some children with autism know the routes to multiple distant destinations. Others display amazing "calendar skills," remembering the day and date of events that occurred months earlier, or figuring out the day of the week of events that occurred before they were born or that will occur in the future, and being skilled at various other processes involving numbers. "Bobby" was one such child. His therapist wrote of this five-year-old boy who had not yet begun school or had any formal instruction:

Although his speech was still idiosyncratic and it was still common for him to run up and down, flapping his arms, he was now able to read, sounding out any words he didn't know; he could add and subtract; his memory was phenomenal, and he could remember many telephone numbers and addresses, as well as the complete New York City bus and subway systems! He could also remember the dates on which events occurred. (Pinney and Schlachter 1983, 233)

A few months later, now six years old, he spent a month in London with his therapist, who had returned there. At that time she noted:

By the time he left he knew by heart the entire London Underground and all the bus routes; sometimes sitting up until three o'clock in the morning, surrounded by pieces of paper, mapping these details and noting the connections. (238)

Furthermore, Bobby could apply this information, although still in ways that may have seemed odd if not bizarre, as another adult reported:

He would stand by the sliding doors; he would announce to the people inside the train what station we had reached and what lines intersected at that station. He would then, when the doors had opened, announce to the people standing outside where the train was going and what lines it would intersect with further along the route. (240)

The developmental psychologist Howard Gardner has proposed a theory of multiple intelligences, which he has presented in publications such as the books *Frames of Mind* and *Multiple Intelligences*. The functioning of people with autism was important in the formation of this theory. While children with autism generally have very poor linguistic or verbal skills, which are commonly equated with intelligence, a substantial number of autistic children undoubtedly have superior ability in the area that Gardner calls spatial intelligence. Other children with autism excel at what Gardner refers to as logical-mathematical intelligence or at what he calls musical intelligence. One recent follow-up study of autistic children found that about a quarter of the individuals studied had a cognitive skill significantly above the mean of both their own overall cognitive level and that of the general population.

"How is my son doing?" a father asks rhetorically in the introduction to his second book about his then eleven-year-old autistic child. "He is doing better than he has done, but not as well as I would have hoped. If I had once seen his malady as transient, I now know it to be permanent. . . . And as for Noah's future—I prefer not to think about it" (Greenfeld 1978, 3).

ADOLESCENCE AND YOUNG ADULTHOOD

In a 1995 letter appealing for contributions, the Autism Society of America reported the following story from a parent of an autistic young adult.

> Last week, I was shopping for a winter coat for my daughter, Stephanie. While we were trying on coats something upset her terribly. Stephanie, who is eighteen and has autism, threw herself on the floor and started kicking, crying, and screaming at the top of her lungs. I pleaded with her to tell me why she was so upset, but nothing I could do would calm her down.

Stephanie's tantrum was wreaking havoc. The sales clerks and customers were staring and whispering and I even heard one woman criticizing my parenting skills.

I wanted to yell to that woman, "Put yourself in my shoes! I'm doing my best here. . . . "

Adolescence may bring an exacerbation of continuing problems, and the appearance of new ones. A small proportion of autistic adolescents have seizures for the first time, and the seizures may be associated with behavioral deterioration—more rituals, compulsions, and aggression. Some mildly disabled adolescents become aware of their social limitations and are greatly distressed by them. Aggressive and self-injurious behavior may become more disruptive and dangerous.

New problems accompanied Ned Christopher's approaching adolescence. Ned began having outbursts of aggressive behavior in which he attacked his mother, pulling at her and pinching her, until she was covered with bruises. More and more he appeared to be in an agitated state, and soon he began lashing out at others. After almost a year of professional help of various kinds that accomplished little, Ned was moved out of his family home. It took six more years of consultation with some of the best professionals in California before Ned's aggressive behavior seemed to fade, but the promise of his early years did not return.

In contrast, the screeching, hitting, biting, and tantrums of some autistic children stop by adolescence, and their rigidity loosens up enough to make everyday living less stressful for them and more tolerable for the family. A very small proportion of youngsters with autism achieve near-normal functioning and are doing well in school, with their disability designation either dropped or changed to indicate a less severe disorder. Others, while still recognized as autistic, may become more socially oriented, and may make progress in academic work while developing greater independence in everyday functioning. The special abilities of some autistic adolescents in such areas as art, music, mathematics, science, or computer science may receive wider recognition and continue to develop during these years.

Special abilities do not necessarily go hand-in-hand with near-normal functioning. Clara Park's daughter Jessy, whose development was referred to in chapter 1, showed giftedness in mathematics as well as great skill in art, but in adolescence and young adulthood, in spite of an IQ in the average range, some of her thinking was like that of a child. She had great difficulty, for example, in dealing with language on anything but a literal level. In her early twenties Jessy was working at understanding proverbs, a major project for her. In trying to master the proverb "Don't cross that bridge until you come to it," she asked: "Does it mean go over the bridge or go under?" And in applying this proverb to a real situation when she thought the family cat was lost but it later showed up, she said: "And there wasn't any bridge!" Some months later when Jessy caught herself obsessing about threatening clouds she said: "It would be crossing the bridge too early—I would fall into the water" (Park 1986, 95).

Literalness in language is a feature very commonly found in children, adolescents, and adults with autism. A mother reported the following episode involving her son:

> After several years of hard work with my son Michael, he was finally doing fairly well fitting into the community.
> For his eleventh birthday I took him with me to the bakery to let him order his cake himself, with the cartoon characters he preferred. He did real well answering questions like what flavor, color frosting, filling. . . . You could tell he was losing patience, though, when the lady asked him what he wanted the cake to say.
> He glanced up at her and said, "Are you crazy! Cakes can't talk! (Gilpin 1993, 4–5)

Another parent's tale of literal language is as follows:

> Our family Saturday project was to scrub oil spills off the driveway. I'd just gotten started when I had to go back inside for another bucket of water. When I returned, I found my son, who has autism, scrubbing merrily away while he was holding his face close to the stain and yelling at the top of his lungs. At first I was totally confused, until I noticed the detergent we were using, Shout. You've guessed it, he was following their slogan and was trying to "Shout it out!" (Gilpin 1994, 62)

Ted, an autistic young adult who had overcome most of his communication problems, also treated words literally. When his mother asked him the meaning of "a bum steer," a phrase he had read aloud from a bill-board, Ted replied: "That's a cow without a job." He became quite upset at the ensuing laughter. It turned out that on an earlier occasion Ted had asked someone about this billboard and had been answered with the pun he had just repeated. Ted had not recognized that the response he had received was meant as humor (Hart 1989, 278). He, in fact, wanted very much to have a sense of humor but couldn't grasp the basic charac-teristics of humor, the qualities of jokes that make them funny. He worked at it, creating "knock, knock" jokes like the following: "Knock, knock." "Who's there?" "Ms." "Ms. who?" "Ms. Brutal Gorilla!" He would follow his joke with the question, "Funny?" (288). Ted couldn't tell what others would find humorous.

For many individuals with autism, adults as well as children, nothing about language comes easily. It's almost as if an innate capacity of hu-mans to acquire language naturally is damaged or missing in autism, and every aspect of language has to be learned separately through delib-erate study. Even when people with autism are strongly motivated and work hard, like Jessy Park and Ted Hart, the process of developing nor-mal language skills may be painstakingly slow.

I met Melvin P. at a conference of a state association on autism. He had been singled out to receive an award for his accomplishments. He was a student at a junior college who had good course grades that he achieved by dint of very hard work. He read a brief speech of thanks for the award and returned to his seat, searching his mother's face for feedback on how he had done. When the session ended people were standing around talking, and I noticed that Melvin P. was standing alone. I introduced myself to him and began a conversation.

"Mr. P. I was happy to hear that you're doing so well at college."
[*A long time passes with no response even though Mr. P. is looking at me. I again attempt to initiate a conversation, this time providing a question that should be easy for him to answer.*]

"What courses are you taking at college?"

"Computers. I'm a computer major."
[*Long pause*]

"How many credits are there in that program?"

"I don't know."

[*Long pause*]

"What other kinds of courses do you take?"

"Math. Communications."

[*Long pause*]

"Is the semester over?"

"It ended on May 18."

[*Long pause*]

"Are you going to summer school?"

"I'm going again in September. I have to ask my counselor how many credits the program has."

[*Long pause*]

"How many credits did you take this semester?"

"Twelve. Thank you for talking to me."

At that point Melvin P. seemed to need a break from the effort involved in his role in the conversation. It was none too soon; I too needed a break from the effort my role had involved. The long pauses in the conversation occurred because I was waiting for Mr. P. to elaborate on his short factual responses, or ask me a question, or introduce a new idea, all strategies for maintaining a conversation. I wondered about his conversations with peers who were very likely of greater interest to him but who could not be counted on to keep supplying him with questions. Could Mr. P. maintain a conversation without being cued by questions? Could he contribute enough to a conversation to engage the interest of other young adults who were not autistic? Could he "mind-read" them well enough to tell when someone was interested?

The end of schooling, which comes at twenty-one years of age for most individuals with autism, often marks the beginning of a difficult transition period. First, everyday routines are disrupted, and any major change is stressful to people with autism. There is also the question of what is to take the place of school. Few autistic adults go on to college, and few can move into jobs independently. Since 1991 transition planning has been a required component of educational programs for older adolescents with significant disabilities. When school programs and state supported programs for adults with developmental disabilities are well coordinated, a twenty-one-year-old with autism will immediately move into a supported work program in the community or a sheltered work program operated by a disability agency. Unfortunately, significant problems frequently occur in this process, and the movement to work is rarely smooth.

The other issue that often arises at about this point in the lives of autistic individuals is where they will live. By the time the person with autism reaches young adulthood, most parents and other family caregivers feel totally exhausted. Some parents may be approaching their late years and feel their energies and health deteriorating. Others may feel that after twenty-one years, they need a chance to experience the freedom common to other parents whose children have grown up. Thus, many families begin to look for another place or way of living for their son or daughter. While many supervised and supported living alternatives have become available since the early 1980s, making a good match between the needs or desires of the autistic individual and his family on the one hand and the available residential arrangements on the other, frequently proves to be a time-consuming and stressful process.

I am writing this chapter after returning from a visit to a group home and a day program for autistic adults. The agency providing these services is operated by two members of the family of an autistic man. I first met one member of this team many years earlier, when we were both on an advisory panel on services for siblings of individuals with developmental disabilities. Today, this sibling serves as my guide.

Our starting point is a retail shop that features handicrafts by autistic adults, in addition to other items. The adults producing these items are at work in one section of the shop. Scattered about the store are tiny signs reading, Your Purchase Helps Our Autistic Young Adults To Be Productive . . . And Employed. It's close to Christmas so many of the products featured reflect that seasonal theme—decorated wreaths and linens embroidered with Christmas motifs. Also displayed are items not tied to the seasons, like note cards. I buy a box of these cards, drawn by their charming young look and humor. Marshall, the brother of my guide, is the artist on several of them. He is a productive person. For five hours each day he works at tasks involved in creating various items for sale. Marshall still sometimes exhibits behavior that causes stress to people who love him and may frighten some people who don't. Although he usually communicates through speech, at times when he's very upset he might make sounds like loud barking and hit his thigh with his clenched hands. During my visit I happen to witness one such episode. Afterwards Marshall takes my hand and strokes it while telling me about computer games he likes — almost as if he wants to make sure I experience the gentle, loving side that's very much a part of him.

It's easy, when you focus on young children as I had been doing, to fall into the trap of thinking that if only autistic children could achieve language and communication, they would be on their way to near-normal functioning. Not so, the adults I saw today reminded me. The nine adults in the shop all spoke; however, how they spoke and what they said was still quite unusual. Daniel is a man I met in the shop. He lives in an apartment with another autistic man as his roommate, under the supervision of the agency providing the services and programs I was observing. In his forties now, his need for control over his environment has taken on an obsessive-compulsive quality. Not only does Daniel speak, he talks incessantly, relating every detail of situations or episodes that concerned him. Daniel works alone, because when he works with others he becomes so involved in explaining his concerns that he totally ignores his work tasks. Cognitively Daniel is capable of much more than he is doing, but a way of harnessing his intelligence into work consistent with his capabilities has not yet been found. Community work positions are being developed for some of the adults in the programs. Whether Daniel will be one of them is questionable.

At this point a good-looking man of about forty enters the shop and delivers something to the agency director. I'm not sure whether he is an autistic man or a staff member. He quietly beckons me to his side. "I'm very interested," he says in a soft voice, "in knowing whether you were born in Manhattan."

After I answer affirmatively, he continues. "What hospital were you born in?"
I give its name. "What was the date of your birth? I'm just interested," he
states, trying to assure me that he means no harm by this question. At this
point I am rescued by my guide. "It's not appropriate to ask people that ques-
tion when you've just met them," my interrogator is told.

Another man starts to talk to my guide about his daily trips to the shop.
He travels independently by train and bus from another part of the city. With
his long hair, laborer-type work clothes, and sturdy physique he looks less like
an easy mark for muggers than most people in this city. But his voice does not
match his appearance. It would frighten off no one. Its high pitch is unex-
pected and has almost a whining quality. The words emerge slowly. This man
has been expelled from several previous programs because of periodic aggres-
sive episodes. Here he has worked out a way to avoid them. Jim can now recog-
nize when he is losing control, announces that he is leaving, and leaves. He is
becoming much better at self-management.

There is also the man I didn't see because he is no longer at the group
home. What I see instead are the plastered walls of what had been his room.
He had punched big holes through two of the walls. Now he was the client of
another agency, one that took the adults with whom other agencies could not
cope. This man too could communicate.

Language is a critical achievement, but language alone doesn't turn
autistic children into nonautistic adults. There are other fundamental
differences in functioning, and significant problems continue to separate
most adults with autism from "typicals."

A monthly meeting of a local chapter of the Autism Society of America
featured a pianist. In fact, the meeting was primarily a concert, and the
concert artist was a young man with autism. It is the evening of the
meeting. We are told that he will play two pieces by Debussy and two
other classical pieces. No music is in sight, but none is needed. He appears to have perfect concentration and plays with a high level of skill.
Having completed this part of his program, he bows, smiles, and takes
a seat in the audience. His mother says something to him, following
which he returns to the piano and announces, "The pop stuff will be

now." He begins with a selection from the Broadway show *Cats* and then continues without interruption through a long medley of show tunes, in the process giving the impression that he could continue indefinitely. He seems very pleased with the enthusiastic response of the audience, even though only about twenty people are present, and several of them are family members or friends.

The pianist's mother then relates some of the details of his development, including his multiple tantrums each day during early childhood; his echolalic and then rote speech; his inability to eat solid food until age seven; the many schools he attended as his parents continued to search for better help; and his ability to play Mozart concertos before he was five although he could not read music and had not yet received any formal instruction. It was not until his junior high school years that this special ability began to help him gain social success, as he became the star of the school orchestra even though he was in a special education class. His mother is obviously proud of him and proud of her own perseverance and determination in fighting against his autism. She summarizes his accomplishments: He drives a car, lives in his own apartment, works professionally as a pianist, has a pet, and has friends.

Then there is some time for questions. Would he care to tell us when language and people started to make sense to him, I ask the pianist. His father, sitting next to him, appears to be helping him with the question. Then the pianist stands up and responds: "My music and language came to me a long time ago, and there's no limit." Afterwards his mother adds: "He's still learning; there are still gaps." Yet the pianist has friends, apparently good ones. Some are there at his concert. His face lights up when he goes to greet them, and they regard him with obvious warmth. He lives independently and he works at what he loves. Recovered from autism? Not completely. But many would envy his life.

4 Families

Nobody can destroy a family quite like

some autistic children . . .

(Hundley 1971, 87)

What is often stolen away by autism is the joy of being a child and the joy of being a parent—the "goodies" that come with having a child, is the way one parent put it. What is lost too is a sense of unlimited potential.

All families go through different stages as children arrive, grow up, and move out, and as parents grow older. Each stage brings new challenges and demands new accommodations. All families experience stresses, and many experience rifts and dislocations. What's particularly different about families in which a child has autism is that the source of momentum for these families, and the fulcrum on which family life turns, is the autistic individual.

Some families fracture from the tension; some grow closer. Some parents experience crisis followed by breakdown, others experience periodic crises and get through them somehow, and still others experience crisis followed by growth. Siblings may be slotted into roles as second-ary parents and teachers. Many are ambivalent about this incursion into their childhood and the scant attention their own needs receive. What-ever the choices family members make and the outcomes of those choices, autism becomes the central experience in their lives for many years, sometimes for a lifetime.

Families can revolve around autism in many ways. Time is one of them. All other interests, activities, and friends not connected to autism get shunted aside, first because of the frantic search for information and a cure, or at least a powerful treatment, later because time is for imple-menting treatment strategies.

Autism also becomes a focal point because of money. It takes lots of it to put comprehensive treatment programs into place. Money becomes an issue: How much of it will it take? Can we manage that? How? If we can't, what do we do next? (Where or to whom do we turn for help?)

Autism is the axis around which the family revolves. Jobs are sacri-ficed, opportunities for advancement are postponed or given up. Fami-lies live apart or uproot themselves altogether from their communities to get their autistic children into better treatment programs, to get them a better chance to be cured. Craig Schulze gave up his job to live in Boston with his autistic son, while his wife and daughter divided their time between Maryland and Massachusetts, because the Boston Higashi school appeared to be his son's best hope, and Jordan needed his family.

Autism may become the nerve center of the family, as when parents are afraid to have additional children lest those children also be autistic, or because it would be unfair to any children to come, or because they couldn't manage other children and their autistic child. Josh Greenfeld reported a conversation he had about his then four-year-old son Noah with Ivar Lovaas of the University of California at Los Angeles, who was supervising Noah's treatment:

> "You worry too much about Noah. You should worry more about your other boy. Or maybe you should have another child. In that way you would worry less. . . . " "But I have eleven children already. To have an autistic child," I said, quoting a Long Island mother of a child like Noah, "is to have ten children." (Greenfeld 1972, 157)

Other children in the family recognize that the autistic child has the spotlight. One sister wrote: "An autistic child in one's midst requires extraordinary compromise for every member of that youngster's family. We all adapt as best we can, but sometimes the penalty for our constant accommodation is considerable" (Zatlow 1982, 50).

Parents of autistic children assume a multitude of roles in addition to those played by parents of typical children. They are searchers in quest of cures, or at least effective treatments. They are advocates, fighting for the services and supports they believe will give their children a better chance for a good life. They are therapists and therapy coordinators. Some parents fill these roles better than others do, but all parents grapple with them.

One mother kept searching until she learned about Landau-Kleffner syndrome and found that her son could benefit from the treatment used for this disorder. Another mother searched until she learned about auditory integration training and found that it improved her daughter's functioning. These were not well-known approaches. Other parents have concluded that one of the better known approaches such as applied behavior analysis is the best one for their child. Still, it took time, energy, and dedication to engage in the search that led to this conclusion.

Some parents, having searched and found what they believe is the most effective treatment currently available, are still driven. The best is not enough. What they seek is a cure, one they hope will help their own son or daughter as well as the children of others. These parents are the force behind many research efforts today. They establish research foundations, make donations to existing institutions for research on autism, prod the research community to focus more attention on autism. Autism continues to be the center of their lives.

Parents are the primary advocates for expanded services to autistic children, adolescents, and adults—their own and the children of others. The 24,000-member Autism Society of America is a parent-founded-and-driven organization. A 1995 parent newsletter from a UCLA clinic that treats children with autism lists seventeen affiliated parent groups around the country. The major function of most of these groups is advocacy. Autism is in the bones of the parents who make up these groups.

Before the advent of federal laws mandating services to young children with disabilities, parents were often their sole teachers or their primary teachers. Many devised and implemented their own home treatment programs. Today parents more commonly act as co-teacher or co-therapist, treatment coordinator, and service monitor. Autism drives their lives.

At times it can become too much. Craig Schulze, unable to halt his son's deterioration and faced with a dramatic sacrifice for his son, underwent a crisis and recognized that he had to heal himself. Lurline Morphett collapsed and briefly wound up in a mental hospital from years of tension accumulated in the process of raising her autistic son.

Fantasies of getting rid of the autistic child may surface. One night Mary Callahan and her husband, driven to the edge by their young son's incessant crying, and rejecting the idea of placing him in an institution, had the following conversation:

> "We could kill him." I was the first to say it.
> "We could," Rich answered, looking down at his hands. "You could get something at work, couldn't you? An injection of something?"
> "Yeah, but it would show up on autopsy. And if the drug didn't, the needle hole would."
> We sat in silence a while longer.
> "He could have an accident, like drowning in the bathtub or something," Rich said. . . .
> "We'd go through life knowing we've killed our own son."
> "We'd know we did it for him."
> "We could never get a divorce," I said. We both laughed hysterically, unable to stop, even when we stopped thinking it was funny.
> We talked for hours, able at last to admit our helplessness to each other. (Callahan 1987, 59)

Sometimes the autistic child may be at acute risk of abuse.

> On the day in question he screeched in my ear just once too often. Something inside me snapped and I temporarily lost control. Suddenly

I hated that child so much that I could not resist hurting him. I slapped him about the head, harder and harder, revelling in the release of my pent up emotions. I could feel them pulsing out of my hands with each blow.

When I eventually regained my composure I was horrified at what I had done. (Morphett 1986, 65)

Parents are not the only family members whose lives revolve around the autistic child. Autistic children are also the center of action in the lives of their sisters and brothers. Letters and other brief pieces by siblings of autistic individuals frequently appear in the newsletter of the Autism Society of America. Most, like the letter that follows, express love for the child with autism, with only passing reference to difficulties (as if it were wrong and bad to dwell on them).

Dear Advocate:

My brother is autistic. It is kind of hard living with him, but he is just like anyone else. I love him very much. I would rather have him as a brother than any other brother in the world. (Nickelsen 1996, 4)

Other statements, often from adult siblings, reveal more complex feelings and relationships.

I always thought it was a trick. . . . This child who tore my hair, who scratched my hands and bit my arms, who broke all my things and scared my friends away. . . . I knew it was just a mean trick and I scratched back, fought back and made him listen to me, because, I said, "you're not special, you're playing a trick and I can see right through you." I made him play with me and I made him copy me. . . . That was many years ago. . . .

I called him today because I love him so much and because I resented him and fought him and protected him for so many years. (Kiebala 1995, 10–11)

The boy who wrote the letter below was encouraged to express his feelings, and he did.

Dear Doctor,

My mom told me to write this letter because I can't come. It's about my sister Hannah. It's hard to live with Hannah, she's almost always mean to me. She bites, kicks, and hits me. . . . None of my friends want to come to my house because they think she's gonna do something to them. . . . Hannah is always bothering me so I get really mad at her. She never gets in trouble. . . . I've gone to lots of shrinks, counselors, and doctors to try and learn about what to do about Hannah, but they never help much. Hannah always gets the attention because my mom is always dealing with Hannah. (Isaiah 1995, 7)

The three letters above mirror common themes heard from siblings. Which type of response pattern is most typical of a sibling probably depends on a variety of factors, some of which parents can't control and some of which they can. An autistic sister or brother is easier to love and teach if she or he doesn't hurt you and doesn't break your cherished possessions. An autistic brother or sister may be easier to play with and teach if you have another brother or sister to help you do this. An autistic sibling may be easier to accept when you feel your parents respect your rights too and understand why you're angry and give you some attention. Recognition of these response patterns doesn't make it easy for parents to change these situations. Lurline Morphett regrets that she did not realize how difficult life was for her nondisabled daughter, but she doesn't know whether she could have made it better even if she had recognized her daughter's strain.

In the preface to her book *Siblings of Children with Autism,* Sandra Harris refers to the needfulness of the sisters and brothers of autistic children: "But when I listen to the voices of these young people in sibling support groups, or in individual conversations, I am struck by the urgency of their needs." Harris describes one mother who kept the needs of her nondisabled son in the picture while she coped with her autistic daughter.

My seven-year-old daughter who has autism broke one of her brother's favorite toys the other day. He was upset and wanted me to punish her. At first I thought it wouldn't do any good, but then I realized that even if she didn't learn anything, he would feel that I was standing up for him, and it would make him feel better. So, I sent her to her room. (Harris 1994, 97)

Why do some families who have an autistic child appear to fare better than others? For a multitude of reasons, some of them related to the nature of the child's characteristics and some existing independent of it. Almost all parents of children with significant disabilities experience high levels of stress during some periods of their son or daughter's development. Stress may come from grief, from exhaustion, from not seeing progress, from fear for the child's future, from anger over what is being sacrificed by other family members. Whatever the nature of the child's disability, some families do better than others because they cope better with stressful situations in general. Of course the autistic child or adolescent's characteristics strongly affect the family's ability to cope. It is more difficult to cope effectively when you see your son injuring himself or hurting his sister or brother. It is harder when your child attacks you often and has prolonged tantrums. It is a formidable task to keep going in the face of periods of deterioration, when your child appears to be going backwards or at best standing still in spite of all your efforts over years. Coping well becomes easier when the autistic child responds in some ways and begins to show signs of learning; when he hurts himself and others less; and when these changes occur while the child is still young. The basically healthy family can then begin to recoup, tend to the needs of other family members, and retrieve the experience of enjoyment.

Families do better when they have strong support networks. Temple Grandin's mother credits her neighbors with helping both Temple and herself. Some families can count on friends, as another mother explains.

> One of my closest friends, Pam, a divorcee with four young children, phoned me one day to make a special request. She said in effect, "I insist that you bring Simon to my house at least once a week, that you continue to do this until he feels at home here. Then you must leave him with me for as long as you wish, and take a break for yourself." Overwhelmed to the point of tears I gratefully accepted her suggestion, and as it turned out Pam was one of the few people whom Simon was content to be with, and her youngest son, Jason, became his first playmate. (Morphett 1986, 66)

Other families receive crucial support from a grandparent who has a special relationship with the autistic child or youth, and who provides the family with badly needed periods of respite. Judy Barron reported: "My mother . . . gave much of her attention to Sean. I drove him to her house after school several days a week, and the two of them spent afternoons together" (1992, 175).

When parents can't turn to family or friends, some find two other resources of support helpful. One of these is respite care services, which allow parents to take a break, do something for themselves, or think about the needs of their other children. Many disability agencies provide respite care services, and they may be available at no cost to families. Unfortunately, such services, whether delivered in the family home or at an agency site, can turn out to be disastrous experiences when the respite care worker does not know the autistic child and has not learned how to relate to him productively.

Many parents find that parent support groups are very useful to them. Sharing "disasters" and other experiences, listening to what worked and didn't work for other families, and finding out how other families coped, give some parents a sense of connectedness that they find comforting. In 1996 the Beach Center on Families and Disabilities of the University of Kansas reported that there were over five hundred parent-to-parent support programs in the country, although these programs served parents of children with various disabilities. Some of these programs include one-to-one support, with parents of younger children being matched with experienced, trained parents of older children and adults. Support groups for siblings may also serve valuable functions, but such support groups are less often available.

Arthur was thirty-five years old. His parents, aging and experiencing health problems, could no longer cope with having him at home. In addition, they were terrified of the possibility that Arthur's care would become his younger sister's responsibility. They had lived through Arthur at ages three and four being rejected by all the nursery schools within traveling distance, and at age five being rejected by the public schools; Arthur not beginning to talk until almost age six, by which time his parents despaired of his ever speaking; Arthur needing to be constantly monitored; and Arthur being suspended from special programs. They had somehow dealt with all that and much more, but now, after Arthur had acquired some significant skills—spoke fluently, dressed and groomed himself, could prepare some simple meals, and could engage in a few activities in the neighborhood independently— his parents had almost reached the end of their endurance. Thirty-five years of fear about what might happen next had taken its toll. His constant repetitive questioning grated on them, as his need for sameness restricted their existence. When a new form of problem behavior appeared in their adult son, they couldn't cope with it.

Had Arthur's parents reached this point before the 1980s, the options available to them would have been quite limited; but it was the 1990s, and many more possibilities existed. Arthur's parents began to explore them. A short time later, when a family crisis occurred, respite care services were arranged for Arthur. This was the first time in thirty-five years that Arthur's parents had a break from the continuous care of their autistic son. To their surprise and relief, no major catastrophe occurred during the period of time when Arthur stayed in the home of a couple experienced in working with autistic adults. A year later Arthur was living in a group home and, after an initial difficult period of getting used to this change in his life, Arthur was doing well.

And what of Arthur's parents? Having ordered their lives around Arthur's care for so long, they had to reorient themselves and figure out what to do with their newly found time. After a period of time, they began to enjoy the quiet that had been missing from their home for so long. They now see Arthur on weekends, and he stays over at his family home on special occasions when he chooses to do so. The tension has drained out of the family. As Arthur said over and over again in preparing himself for his move, "I'm a man now. It's time for me to move on." It was that time for his parents too.

We have been focusing on the stress that autism brings into families and the need for family support, but there is another side of this picture— love, devotion, pride, and a sense of purpose. It's easy to see in Wayne

Gilpin, who compiled and published two books—*Laughing and Loving with Autism* and *More Laughing and Loving with Autism*—filled with anecdotes about the adolescent son who lives with him and about the children of other parents whose lives have been enriched by their autistic children. It's there too in the many families in which no one has written a book or spoken at a conference.

No one asks for autism, just as no one asks for cerebral palsy or epilepsy or any other developmental disorder. It happens. We don't know how to prevent autism. We don't know how to cure it. Treatment outcomes vary greatly. Some families are able to create lives of satisfaction even though their sons and daughters have not lost their autism. Ruth Sullivan commented in a recent interview: "Joseph opened up a whole new world for me. . . . It's a cliché, I know, but it's been a wonderful life" (Interview 1995, 15). Perhaps one day soon, when we know more about how to help children with autism, many parents with autistic sons and daughters will be able to respond to Ruth Sullivan's conclusion by saying "ditto."

part two Treating Autism

5 We Have a Dream

What is my dream? My dream is that somehow
Noah slowly improves, and everything else, all
other dreams, are contingent upon that. But how
will he improve?

(Greenfeld 1972, 79)

One evening in April 1995 I caught a train to Westchester so that I could be at a conference on autism early the next morning. It was after 9 P.M. when I arrived at Rye, New York. Only one adult person left the train, an African-American woman carrying a large duffel bag and a boy of about five. When I entered the motel van that arrived a few minutes later, two well-dressed women were already in it. They were talking about their children's treatment programs of six to seven hours a day, whether to leave therapists alone with their children, and whether every treatment session should be videotaped for review by a senior therapist. How long did it take for your son to get used to the sessions? one mother asked. The other mother responded: He pretty much tantrummed for a month. Now he doesn't mind. They work for five minutes and then play for ten. And the therapists—they're in control. They know what the child can do. And the good thing is I can always get a consultation on the phone. It's worth the seventy dollars an hour.

Those two women and I were going to the same conference, "Behavioral Intervention in Autism: Stepping into the Future," as was the woman with the five-year-old who had been at the train station. So was a group of parents from Staten Island whom I knew and now met at the motel. These wives of policemen, firemen, and teachers, and, as I later learned, the African-American mother, were all struggling to provide for their autistic children the kinds of services that the Westchester families already had.

The performing arts center at the State University College at Purchase, with its high ceilings and bi-level design, is spacious, modern, and light. I walked about listening to snatches of conversation while the continental breakfast was being served. "Did you hear about this new book on autism . . . ?" "Someone just lent it to me; I'll read it right after the conference." "Have you made any progress with his toileting? They should be able to get that by age four." "I was desperate. I called my mom and said, 'Mom, can you come for a month; I can't handle this.'"

The orchestra of the thirteen-hundred-seat auditorium is completely filled, as is the balcony as far back as I can see. Mostly women, mainly in their twenties or early to mid-thirties; a few older women who might be grandmothers or professionals. Each of these people has paid a hundred dollars to be there that day, two hundred if they will be there for the next day as well, and a total of three hundred if they reserved a place at the dinner that evening. There's a sense of purpose, excitement, and great importance in the air.

The program begins. *Foundation for Educating Children with Autism, Inc.*, appears on the screen. The president of this Westchester sponsoring organization explains that it was formed by parents in July 1994 to establish schools for young children with autism. The first school is to open in January 1996. The audience is interested but slightly impatient. They have come to see and hear the guru of this movement, O. Ivar Lovaas, professor of psychology at the University of California, Los Angeles.

Ivar Lovaas is of medium height, with gray hair and beard, and a slight accent left over from his Scandinavian background. He is both dramatic and informal. The cause of autism? "We don't have a clue. Probably a multiplicity of etiologies. Autism is a guess. . . . If we all focus on looking for the cause of autism we wind up in a blind alley. You can disagree on whether a child has autism but if you look at behavior, you can plan intervention and measure effectiveness." Seemingly casually he debunks other approaches: Three or four times a year a special treatment for autism is invented; none of them works, he implies. Behavioral therapy doesn't assume a sudden breakthrough. It's a slow, stepwise process.

He illustrates and explains autistic behavior through videotapes, showing children at different points of the treatment process. We watch in fascination and something akin to horror the rocking, twirling, and pacing; the hand flapping and staring at fingers; the turning on and off of lights, the lining up of small objects; and the flicking of a stick. These are self-stimulating behaviors, we are told.

Then comes a more difficult and controversial subject—the treatment of self-abuse, referred to here as self-injurious behavior. The videotapes show children banging their heads against furniture, biting themselves, pulling out their hair, socking themselves. In the 1960s, Lovaas admits, he did use physical punishment to treat this behavior, and shock therapy was sometimes used. While it was effective in the short run, the suppression did not last. We don't use punishment now, he reports. If you ignore the self-injurious behavior it will go up initially, he tells us, but soon the rate will go down. We also reinforce the child for other behaviors every time there is a pause in the self-injurious behavior, he continues.

More videotape, this time Lovaas at the first session with a three-year-old girl. He seats her in a chair facing him, hooking his feet around the chair so that she can't escape. Then he stands her up. She screams but can't go anywhere. As soon as she sits down again he offers her food. She refuses it and begins to tantrum. He pulls her up and then verbally and physically directs her to sit. As soon as she is seated he gives her a glass of soda. She drinks it. Later he no longer has to physically guide her to sit. He pulls her up, tells her to sit, and she does. He substitutes social reinforcers for food. "G-o-o-o-o-o-d," he says, elongating that word immensely, and adding a hug. "Look at me," he adds. She looks and he reinforces her.

"You have to learn to be a bitch," he tells the parents in commenting on the videotaped session. "Say 'sit' in a loud voice; later you can lower it."

Lovaas directs the very full agenda for the rest of the day. He outlines the central features of the treatment program: forty to sixty hours a week plus informal teaching by parents for one to four years if the child recovers; otherwise, for the rest of life. Live videotapes are the high point of the day. Several children have been brought to the conference for demonstrations of the behavioral treatment developed by Lovaas. A therapist works with one child backstage while a simultaneous videotape is being shown on the very large stage screen.

A two-and-one-half-year-old puts blocks into a shape sorter and is reinforced with raisins. Being swung up in the air is used as another reinforcer, as is a few minutes to "go play." "Come here," the therapist says, and then "Good coming," when the child complies. "Sit" and "Good sitting" are coupled with a tiny piece of a Snickers bar. The therapist taps a block on the table when the toddler's attention wanders. This child, we are told, has been in treatment for close to forty hours a week for one month.

The other children are older and have been in treatment longer. A five-year-old is still having difficulty picking out some of the shapes the therapist names. He prompts her, pointing to the correct shape and saying its name. She watches the materials attentively. At one point she uses her right hand to hit her left one. A second therapist appears. "What's your name?" he asks her. She tells him her first name. "What's Momma's name?" She responds correctly. "What's your last name?" Correct again. We are told that this child was in therapy for six months before she said her first name. A year later her vocabulary consists of about 150 words, but she still expresses herself with nonspeech sounds when she is under stress.

Another child is shown reading word cards, writing letters, and writing her name. Her reinforcers are hugs, high fives, "Good girl," and a sense of accomplishment. "I did it," she says with obvious pride, after she wrote a letter the therapist named. "She's on her way to recovery," Lovaas comments.

Tumultuous applause is the response of the audience at the end of the day. This is what they came for—to hear the person who has provided them with hope, who has shown them a way. He has also uttered that word they pray for every day: recovery. This is the dream that brought them here from Kansas and Vermont and Vancouver, the dream of their children having what we think of as a real life. It was what made them clap and cry and then leave exhilarated, with new hope, renewed confidence, and a sense of determination.

What's happening here? Has Ivar Lovaas found the key to recovery from this terrifying disorder? How has he come to be viewed as a savior by so many families? And why now, when he has been doing, and reporting on, behavioral treatment for years? Is recovery from autism really possible?

To answer the "how" and "why now" parts of this enigma, we have to turn to Catherine Maurice. In 1993 a book entitled *Let Me Hear Your Voice* was published. Catherine Maurice was its author, and her two autistic children were its subject. Within a few months, through an article in a popular magazine and word-of-mouth among parents, her book became almost a cult item—the proof and the protocol for recovery. And Catherine Maurice credits Ivar Lovaas with the rescue of her children. It was his work, she writes, that charted a path to the journey home.

Anne-Marie was the second child of Catherine Maurice and her husband, Marc. Like her older brother, she seemed perfectly normal at first, although somewhat somber and a bit too content with solitary play. Her parents thought of her as their shy and sensitive child. Still, she would lift her arms to be picked up as she called out for her daddy, and laugh when he kissed her and tickled her. She would also seek out her mother and gaze at her lovingly. At eighteen months Anne-Marie was silent. Gone was her "hi" and "bye" and approximation of "I love you." A few months later the diagnosis of autism was confirmed. And then, when their third child was little more than eighteen months old, it happened again.

Catherine Maurice is not your typical parent. She has a Ph.D. She writes movingly and convincingly. Her description of initial joy, followed by glints of concern, and then full-blown anxiety about signs that could not be ignored, made parents feel as if they were reliving their own experiences. So when Catherine Maurice communicated her conclusion that the Lovaas approach was the only one that offered a chance of recovery, that she had used it in spite of her initial revulsion at some aspects of this method, and that this approach had saved her children, other parents listened.

The dinner speaker at the Westchester conference on behavioral intervention in autism was Catherine Maurice. She is a slim, rather attractive, dark-haired woman who speaks in a soft and tenuous voice. Both her children had completely recovered, she told the six hundred people who had been lucky enough to get reservations for the dinner. An evaluation had confirmed this. Her daughter was doing well in a third-grade class and her son in the first grade. "For many parents my children represent hope," she told her audience. Yet she also mentioned her "very fragile sense of security about my children."

Stories of individual children or even two of them, case studies if you will, are of great value but they can also be dangerous. What were the critical variables that allowed and enabled Catherine Maurice's children to recover? We don't really know. Would the same approach have led to the same outcomes with different autistic children? We don't really know. Are many parents who try to replicate Catherine Maurice's methods going to be disappointed with the outcomes for their children? Undoubtedly. Should they be discouraged? Should professionals advise them not to expect or hope for this outcome? No. At the Westchester conference on autism I commented to a nurse from Canada on the likelihood that many of the parents there were going to be very disappointed when their children didn't recover. That's not true, she responded. "We've already been so hurt we will accept this—I have two autistic children," she continued, "one retarded and one not retarded. Even if my retarded son doesn't recover, at least I'll know that I've given him the best possible chance I could."

Is this mother right? I asked myself. I was impressed but not totally convinced, and Lovaas left me uncomfortable, uneasy.

I went back to New York City with the African-American woman and her five-year-old son who had arrived on the same train as I had. They were the only black people I saw at the conference. We had begun talking at the dinner table the previous night. The presence of her strikingly beautiful young son had brought her many interested listeners.

Coming to this conference had been a financial strain, she told me, but she would do anything to help her son. How could he survive the way he was? In Brooklyn? In their neighborhood? I asked her about her son's schooling. He had been in a special preschool program for two years, she told me, but it hadn't helped. This year, in a public school class for autistic children, he had gotten worse. "He has an aide assigned to him now because he had started biting," she explained. She had tried to get her son into a class in his school where they did some behavioral training. It was a special program that parents had to volunteer for, but she was told there was no more room in it. "Does he speak at all?" I asked, as I had not heard a sound come from this child who hardly left her arms. "He can talk," she replied. "Sometimes he says something to me, but not so often. Sometimes I work with him at home and he talks."

She was very glad she had come to the conference, this mother told me. She had talked to many people who had promised her help. Five months later I tried to contact that mother to find out whether any of the promised help had materialized, and to find out how her son was doing. After several tries I reached someone who identified herself as the child's sitter. The boy was in the same school program as last year and no help had arrived, she told me after I explained why I was calling; but he was doing a little better now. His mother would call me back the next day, she promised. That call never came. Desperate parents have no time for people who have no real help to offer their child. This mother had the same dream for her child as did the mothers from Westchester and those from Staten Island. What was different were the resources she could marshal in the struggle to achieve that dream.

TODAY AND YESTERDAY

Hope and expectations have a way of winding down with time, when outcomes don't match dreams. The father of a recently diagnosed two-year-old attended a meeting of a local chapter of the Autism Society of

America. He will not go there again, he told his family. Those people accept their children's autism. He will never accept autism. He will fight it until his son recovers. He will never stop fighting it.

Yet thirty years ago this national organization was founded by a group of fighters. Their dream too was to defeat autism, in their own children and in others'. The organizing meeting took place in Teaneck, New Jersey, in November 1965. About sixty people were present. "We fell on each other," recalls Ruth Sullivan, one of the parents present. "It was heady. For the first time we had hope. . . . It was the most electrifying meeting I have ever been at in my life" (Warren 1984, 102).

In 1969 the fledgling organization had its first annual conference. That too was an exciting and exhilarating meeting with impressive people, including parents who went on to develop programs, serve as consultants, and write books about their personal experiences with autism. Glimmers of current issues or preludes to them pervaded that conference, along with goals now achieved. Ivar Lovaas was the luncheon speaker at the second conference, in 1970, his subject the "Strengths and Weaknesses of Operant Conditioning Techniques for the Treatment of Autism." His message, however, was quite different then: "The program does not turn out normal children, and should a child become normal as we treat him, then that no doubt, is based on the fact that he had a lot going for him when he first started treatment" (Park 1971, 39).

Recovery was not the theme of that conference twenty-five years ago, but the possibility of a life of near-normal functioning was. Mothers spoke with both pride and sadness of the achievements and continuing limitations of their adult children, still odd men out, still struggling to understand and be accepted in the social world.

Now let's fast-forward to 1995 again, this time to July and Greensboro, North Carolina. It is the 1995 national conference of the Autism Society of America. The electricity of the organizing meeting thirty years earlier is gone. Missing also is the fervor of the Westchester meeting that took place three months earlier. Lovaas is not on the program; nor was he on the program in 1994. There is little talk of recovery here. Improvement, programs, strategies, support for families, and recognition of adults with near-normal functioning appear to be the themes.

One of the general sessions is a panel report from an autism research symposium of the National Institutes of Health. A member of the audience asks a question about recovery. A distinguished psychiatrist on the panel replies that in his contact with over eight hundred individuals with autism he has never seen a person who has recovered. What he has seen is symptom remission with near-normal functioning.

This conference does not celebrate recovery or use it as a goal. Too many parents in this organization had been forced to give up this dream. There is Craig Schulze, presenter on a parent panel, the author of *When Snow Turns to Rain*, the story of his son's deterioration and his unsuccessful attempts to reverse it. And Connie Post, also on that panel and the author of two books of poetry about her autistic son, who was placed in a residential center at age six because the family was disintegrating under the barrage of his attacks on his mother and himself. And Clara Claiborne Park, a third panelist, author of the book *The Siege,* about the childhood of her autistic daughter Jessy, whom no miracle has transformed. You wouldn't have to observe Jessy for five minutes to know she's autistic, Clara Park stated at an earlier session. Recovery, when it is mentioned here at all, is referred to quietly.

The major question in my mind after the contrast of these two 1995 conferences is whether the still autistic, obviously impaired adult sons and daughters of many participants at the North Carolina conference would have been different, closer to normal or recovered, if they had been treated with Lovaas's behavioral program when they were young. Or, will most of the children of parents at the Westchester conference still be autistic and obviously impaired in their functioning fifteen or twenty years from now? Have we been shown a way to rescue substantial numbers of children from the devastating effects of autism? Or were the two conferences highlighting different points in the life cycle of autistic individuals and their families?

6 Is Lovaas the Only Game in Town? Intervention Programs for Autistic Children

Autism can be an implacable foe, as anyone who has struggled against it knows. What makes the battle particularly grueling is that the contours of this foe are shadowy; it takes on different shapes with different children and within the same child at different ages. And this foe holds children in a vise-like grip. To wage a successful battle against such an adversary takes fierce determination, and for many children the struggle has no end. Moreover, the battle cannot be waged by professionals alone or parents alone. It takes the combined efforts of a dedicated family, skilled professionals, and a child who (eventually) demonstrates the will and means to fight. The mother of the cum laude university graduate referred to in chapter 2 recalled: "I thought of my son as the count of Monte Cristo, slowly tunneling his way out of autism."

There is no standard treatment for autism. There is instead a history of supposed "breakthroughs" or "miraculous treatments" that turn out not to be miraculous and help only a small proportion of autistic

84

children. In recent years behavioral programs have acquired primacy, and because of Catherine Maurice's story about her recovered children many parents are acting almost as if this approach had miraculous therapeutic power. Lovaas and other skilled educators know better. The story of "recovery" told by Catherine Maurice may appear to be a miracle, they would say, but it is a result of intensive one-to-one work every day over a substantial period of time, starting when the child is very young; and while this sometimes achieves very good results, it doesn't "work" with all children.

Most people want neat solutions to problems. When I teach the introductory course in special education at Hunter College I try to help students see the complexity of many educational issues. One day, after a two-hour class session on the topic of inclusion of children with disabilities in mainstream programs, a student raised her hand and asked: "Well, is inclusion good or bad?" My answer to that question was that there are more useful ways of thinking about this question, like What are the potential benefits and pitfalls of this strategy? What can be done to increase the likelihood that it will be a valuable experience? How do alternate strategies compare in terms of potential benefits and pitfalls? These are the kinds of questions that need to be part of our thinking about any proposed approach or strategy, whether for an individual child with autism or for children with autism in general. And in the end, values play a significant role in selecting educational treatment approaches, particularly when no approach can promise the outcome that is the dream of all parents.

At the present time most forms of treatment for autism are probably best thought of as facilitative, that is, they may pave the way for improved functioning but do not eliminate the core features of autism. They include "alternative" treatments like auditory integration training, which may be facilitative for some children. Megavitamin therapy, dietary treatment, and sensory integration therapy might all be viewed as possibly facilitative interventions for some autistic children. Few, if any, professionals are suggesting such treatments in lieu of educational treatment approaches, and most parents are using them as supplements to such programs. Drug treatment too is at present largely facilitative (at best). The drugs currently being used to treat individuals with autism do not eradicate core characteristics of autism, although they may reduce undesirable behavior like hyperactivity, aggression, and self-injury. Moreover, none of these treatments is entirely without possibly harmful side effects. Drugs may reduce alertness or result in intensified behavioral disturbances whose source is not recognized because they occur after a period of improved functioning on a particular medication. Megavitamin treatment has been reported to cause diarrhea in some children. Auditory integration training may result in a temporary period of increased behavioral disturbance. Therefore, such treatments should be undertaken with thoughtfulness and caution.

In the future we may identify one or more treatment approaches that significantly reduce or even eliminate the core features of autism in a substantial number of children. In the meantime educational treatment remains for most autistic children the most effective approach available; and perhaps the greatest danger in the use of alternative interventions is that they may distract parents from their efforts to identify the best educational approach for their child and ensure that it is implemented with the necessary intensity.

Temple Grandin gives much of the credit for her good functioning to early school experiences.

> At age two and a half I was enrolled in a nursery school for speech-handicapped children. It was staffed by an older, experienced speech therapist and another teacher. Each child received one-to-one work with the therapist while the teacher worked with the other five children. The teachers there knew how much to intrude gently into my world to snap me out of my daydreams and make me pay attention. Too much intrusion would cause tantrums, but without intervention there would be no progress. . . . I would tune out, shut off my ears. (Grandin 1995, 96)

About three years later Temple Grandin began attending a small mainstream kindergarten class in an elementary school.

Temple Grandin's early schooling had many elements that are generally considered optimal today. She began receiving services before age three. She received one-to-one instruction in language. The teaching staff intruded into her autistic world and interrupted her stereotyped activities, but they did so gently. And after receiving intensive special education services before age five, Temple Grandin moved to a mainstream educational program by kindergarten age. In addition to school services Temple Grandin had an excellent home-based program thanks to the governess who kept Temple and her younger sister busy with games and art projects and taught them to skate, play ball, and jump rope, all the while enticing Temple into staying connected to the real world.

What do we know about educational treatment for young autistic children, and what questions or issues still exist? There is virtually no disagreement about the value of early educational intervention. Over twenty years of data collected by federally funded educational projects for children under age five with various developmental disabilities point to this conclusion, as do several studies of programs specifically designed for autistic children. Sandra Harris and her associates at the Douglass Developmental Disabilities Center of Rutgers University found that one year of intensive educational (behavioral) treatment during the preschool years could narrow the gap in IQ and language that separates most autistic children from their normally developing peers.

There is also widespread agreement that educational intervention needs to be intensive if it is to make a significant difference in the functioning of many autistic children. "Intensive" refers to the number of hours a day and week of intervention, the amount of time directly focused on the individual child's learning during those hours, and the duration of weeks, months, or years during which the intervention continues. Lovaas found that ten hours a week of one-to-one behavioral intervention is not enough, while forty hours a week often is. Forty hours is what most parents of young autistic children want; thirty to forty hours is what many professionals believe may be essential in helping autistic children achieve as close to normal functioning as is possible through educational treatment. However, one study that partially replicated the Lovaas Young Autism Project model found that even an average of twenty hours a week of one-to-one behavioral intervention over a period of one year was associated with significant improvement in mental age in close to half of the sample of fourteen children receiving these services (Anderson et al. 1987); and another study found that four out of nine children receiving an average of twenty-nine hours of behavioral intervention a week for two years showed substantial improvement on IQ, language, and adaptive behavior (Birnbrauer and Leach 1993). Neither of these studies reported any children who met the criteria used by Lovaas to define normal behavior or recovery, although the period of intervention in the Anderson study might have been too short to be relevant to the issue of achieving "normal functioning."

There is general agreement that the young autistic child must be helped to become more responsive to his or her environment, particularly to the people in it, but it is here that approaches begin to diverge rather sharply. If we look at how different programs handle initial encounters with children, this point of divergence becomes clear. Some programs use forceful means of intruding into the child's autistic world, while others rely on a combination of enticement and gentle intrusion.

In programs based on or derived from the Lovaas Young Autism Project model, intrusion begins immediately. The initial program objectives usually call for getting the child to attend to the therapist ("Look at me"), follow simple directions ("Sit down; stand up"), and imitate actions modeled by the adult (Taylor and McDonough 1996). Directions are often given in a loud voice. Physical guidance is used to ensure that the child follows the adult's directions, with food or other rewards being used to reinforce the child's compliance. Some young children cry and seek to escape from their instructional sessions for days or even weeks as they are initiated into treatment programs. Catherine Maurice experienced this forcefulness as she watched her daughter being initiated into her behavioral program:

> As soon as Bridget placed Anne-Marie in the opposite chair the crying broke out in earnest. Anne-Marie tried to get out of the chair; Bridget kept placing her firmly back in. She collapsed on the floor; Bridget picked her up and put her back in the chair. She tried to put her hands in front of her face; Bridget took them down and held them in her lap.
>   Anne-Marie was terribly fearful and distraught. She turned and

looked directly at me, for the first time in weeks. Her mouth was trembling.

I was cold and clammy with tension. Was this right? Was I doing the right thing? But I had wanted an assault. Hadn't I decided that we were going to "drag" Anne-Marie out of autism? (Maurice 1993, 87)

This starting point not only paves the way for later program objectives such as imitation of speech sounds but also establishes a pattern for child/therapist interactions: the adult directs, models, and reinforces; the child responds with imitation and compliance. Lack of attention and stereotyped activities ("self-stims," in Lovaas shorthand) are often responded to with sharpness.

In commenting on early intervention strategies, Temple Grandin remarked that while she was one of the autistic children who could be jolted into attention by her teachers, other autistic children would withdraw or collapse altogether in the face of sharp intrusion into their autistic world. Donna Williams was one example of such a child mentioned by Temple Grandin.

Recently, modifications have appeared in behavioral programs to reduce the stress experienced by some young children at the beginning of treatment. Lovaas no longer insists on eye contact at the beginning of his program. He acknowledges that building eye contact is more difficult than he initially conceived and that pressing for it early in the treatment process may be counterproductive with some children. He is also now using physical contact with the mother as a reinforcement during sessions at the beginning of treatment with those children for whom separation from the mother is very stressful.

Most nonbehavioral approaches reject forceful intrusion as counterproductive to the goal of motivating the child to want to interact with others, as do some newer models of applied behavior analysis. Programs that favor enticement of the child into more interaction usually begin quite differently. The adult usually takes his or her lead from the child's behavior, attempting to expand the child's interest in interaction. At the start of treatment the adult may match the child's actions or join in the child's activity focus. This horrifies many behaviorists who are

intent on eliminating the autistic child's stereotyped behavior and eliciting attention to adult directives. Yet mirroring of the child's behavior
as a way of capturing his attention and facilitating interaction is not
without support from research.

Mutual imitation is characteristic of the interactions of infants and
their mothers, and research with young autistic children by Geraldine
Dawson and others shows that when the adult imitates the child's behavior, the child displays more social responsiveness, for example, increased eye contact, touching, vocalizing, and toy exploration. Dawson
speculates that allowing the child rather than the adult to lead the interaction enables the child to regulate the amount of stimulation received
from the other person, thus avoiding painful overstimulation. Behaviorists and others might ask: why should the normal process of mutual
imitation that failed the autistic child in infancy work now? Dawson
reasons that this strategy may be effective if it is provided in megadoses
and is simplified for the child by the elimination of distracting environmental stimuli.

Stanley Greenspan (1992a, 1997) is probably the leading theorist in
the area of developmentally based therapeutic intervention with young
children. His followers include many psychologists, teachers, social
workers, speech/language therapists, and occupational therapists involved in working with children from infancy through the early childhood years. Greenspan, too, believes in intrusion into the world of the
child he refers to as having a multisystem developmental disorder, a
term roughly equivalent to pervasive developmental disorder; but to
Greenspan the intrusion must be congruent with the child's behavior
and must focus on the child's affect. Follow the child's lead, join in, and
expand what the child is doing, he says. The first goal of such intervention is shared attention and engagement. If a child is avoidant,
Greenspan advocates being persistent in pursuit but playful.

Barry Prizant, a communication disorders specialist on the faculty
of Emerson College who has extensive experience with young autistic
children, also uses a developmental approach and believes in enticing
young children into interaction. He delineates a number of "Intervention Strategies to Entice Communication" that includes the following:

Place desired objects so that they are visible to the child but out of the child's reach or in containers that the child needs help opening.

Engage the child in an activity that necessitates a utensil, then withhold the utensil or "sabotage" the function of the utensil.

Offer the child items that the child does not like or that the child does not need for an activity he or she is engaged in.

Set up a turn-taking routine for three or more turns until the child anticipates the steps and then violate a step in the routine. (Prizant and Wetherby 1989, 13)

Let's look at some illustrations of how the treatment of very young children with autism or pervasive developmental disabilities not otherwise specified (PDD/NOS) may differ in programs with different approaches. Melinda entered the Karen Horney Therapeutic Nursery at age three-and-one-half. She had difficulties in relating, poor receptive language, and speech that was largely echolalic. She had areas of competence, too. She could recognize numbers, letters, and colors, and name some objects. Melinda was also hyperlexic. She could "read" (name) the words in children's books without understanding the meaning of what she was reading.

Melinda's teacher began the treatment program by trying to develop reciprocal play with her. The teacher and Melinda took turns blowing bubbles, playing peek-a-boo in front of a mirror, and throwing a ball back and forth. They worked on strengthening Melinda's relationship to her mother through visits to the parents' room during the school program, by using photographs of her mother in the classroom, and by making frequent references to "Mommy." The teachers drew pictures of Melinda at various activities, creating story books by adding written descriptions of what Melinda was doing in each picture. They also put together books of photographs of Melinda and other people in her life. Staff used simple, functional language with Melinda and tried to elicit the same from her. Melinda appeared to become more attached to her mother and more aware of herself. Her speech began to reflect her preferences, for example, "I want bike." "I want cracker." She also began to initiate dramatic play (Koplow et al. 1996).

Nelson was not yet two, but he made no attempt to communicate.

His mother wasn't taking any chances because Nelson's four-year-old brother was autistic, and Nelson had been tentatively diagnosed as having a pervasive developmental disorder not otherwise specified (PDD/NOS). I watched this tiny boy and the young woman who had been his teacher for one month work within a behavioral format in a center-based class for toddlers. They sat facing each other on childsize chairs. Nelson's teacher was trying to get him to imitate her actions. "Hands up," she said as she raised her arms. Nelson lifted his arms and was rewarded with a cheese doodle. Clapping hands was next, and another cheese doodle followed. Then the teacher blew soap bubbles toward Nelson, saying "bubble," "bubble," with an emphasis on the *b* sound, while Nelson watched. Some gentle tickling came next, and Nelson laughed out loud. "Look at me," the teacher said, holding a raisin in front of her face. It was again time for hands up, but this time Nelson rejected the cheese doodle, and his teacher quickly substituted a toy piano designed for toddlers. Nelson cautiously pushed the keys. When bubble time arrived again Nelson went after a large one, broke it, and laughed.

The teacher changed activities. She pulled Nelson up from his chair and then told him to sit down. When he did this, the teacher gave him either a raisin or an opportunity to play briefly with a toy. After this pull up–sit down routine was repeated three times, Nelson began to cry. The teacher stopped, comforted Nelson briefly, and repeated the pull up–sit down exercise once more. Then it was time for a break, and after Nelson found that he couldn't open the room door, he did some jumping and ball throwing with assistance from his teacher.

What had Nelson learned? That if he imitated his teacher's actions and did what she told him to, he would get things he liked to eat and interesting toys to play with. He seemed to have grasped the idea of imitation and may have been in the process of learning to understand some simple verbal phrases. He also seemed to relate well to his teacher, allowing her to provide him with comforting and fun. This instructional session was a far cry from some of the harsh interactions that used to be common in behavioral programs and that still take place in some behavioral programs today. Nelson, however, made it easy to avoid harshness. He made no attempt to hurt anyone, displayed few stereo-typed behaviors, and was easy to reach.

The Language and Cognitive Development Center of Boston, which has been treating autistic children for over twenty-five years, uses a treatment approach that combines developmental and cognitive strate-gies in often inventive ways to entice the child into interaction and en-gagement. The focus of treatment is on expanding the child's behavior and interactions with others. Jack, a two-and-one-half-year-old with au-tism, sat on his mother's lap at the beginning of treatment. Jack was handed pictures of animals one at a time every four or five seconds before he could lose interest or throw the picture. But before receiving the next picture, Jack had to drop the one in his hand into a nearby jar. Initially his mother helped him with this task. Then Jack and his mother were moved to a table, with Jack on one side and his mother on the other. Jack's mother then sent the animal pictures to him in a toy truck that she rolled across the table. Now Jack had to insert the picture he was holding into a slot on the lid of the jar in order to get the next picture. A few sessions later Jack had to send a picture by truck back to his mother. When his mother received the picture, she would hold it up and name all the parts of the animal. At a later point a toy barn with animal figures was introduced; human figures were added afterwards. Through such a process Jack's interests, social interactions, and commu-nication were expanded substantially within six months.

Each of the treatment approaches illustrated in the examples pre-sented here appeared to be effective with the particular child with whom it was used. Would they have been effective with other types of children—older at the start of treatment, more severely impaired, more difficult to interest in any kind of interactive activity? Would they have been as effective if the three children had been switched around, with Jack going to the therapeutic nursery, Melinda to the behavioral pro-gram, and Nelson to the language and cognitive center? Perhaps not, although these are not questions we can answer with a high degree of certainty.

Children who start treatment at the Language and Cognitive Devel-opment Center before age three, as Jack did, have significantly better outcomes with this approach than do those who begin treatment later, according to the center's directors. And while the Language and Cognitive Development Center reports that 48 percent of the children it treats "have returned to their regular public schools able to mainstream in some or all of the classes," these data are referred to as providing only "a rough measure of the Center's effectiveness" (Miller and Eller-Miller 1989, 496). Traditional therapeutic nursery programs are likely to be more effective with children like Melinda who have some language skills than for autistic children with little receptive or expressive language. In fact, with some children like Melinda, therapeutic nursery programs—which focus on spontaneous functional communication and age-appropriate play—may be more effective at nurturing these skills than behavioral programs. And yet it is hard to judge to what extent Melinda's good progress was typical or common, because therapeutic nursery programs usually report effectiveness data only in the form of case studies.

It is frequently said that young children with autism need structure. This argument is often used against preschool special education programs with a developmental approach, against individual therapeutic intervention based on a developmental model like Stanley Greenspan's, and against programs that identify themselves as therapeutic nurseries, all of which are often lumped together and dismissed by parents who have invested all their faith in the Lovaas model. "So-called therapeutic nurseries are not appropriate for autistic children; they are just a waste of time," I've heard parents say, sometimes with a combination of disdain and anger. What all these developmentally based models do share is the belief that the child should have a significant role in selecting and directing his or her own activities, with the adult serving as co-director, model, facilitator, source of support, and environmental engineer. Play and functional learning have central roles in these approaches.

The therapeutic nursery model has existed for many years and was originally designed to serve children considered emotionally disturbed. Children diagnosed as PDD/NOS or autistic are often served in these programs. The curriculum used in therapeutic nurseries is generally rich, and harshness finds no place there. The traditional thera-peutic nursery has as its foundation a combined developmental-psychodynamic approach highly consistent with Stanley Greenspan's approach, and the key dynamic is nurturance—nurturance of a sense of self and nurturance of expression through communication and engage-ment in play. While this approach may be wonderful for some children with PDD/NOS who can understand speech and have begun to com-municate, it may not do well with more severely impaired autistic chil-dren. (Some programs that keep the "therapeutic nursery" title incorpo-rate additional strategies, including behavioral programming, into their models.)

I observed an autistic boy who was almost five in one therapeutic nursery. He was sitting in a sandbox filling a bucket and then pouring the sand out or letting it slip through his fingers, much as Temple Grandin used to do on the beach when she was very young. Another child sat no more than two feet away from him, but he appeared not to notice her. An assistant teacher tried to join his play, to expand it. The boy moved to another area of the room. What he did allow the teacher to do was hold his hands as he jumped up and down on a mini-trampoline, and his smile confirmed that this was something he en-joyed; but what else was he getting out of this preschool experience? What kept going through my head as I watched him was that he would soon be five, had no system of communication, appeared to have little understanding of speech, largely avoided interaction, and engaged in stereotyped play activities. There had to be a better option for him, I kept thinking.

The educational treatment approach receiving the most attention to-day is a behavioral approach or what is frequently referred to as applied behavior analysis. As we noted in chapter 5, many parents of young children are clamoring for such programs in the belief that they hold the key to their child's recovery. What do we mean when we say that the approach used in a particular program is behavioral or uses applied behavior analysis? A simple explanation of a behavioral treatment approach is that it is based on two principles of learning: children will increasingly engage in behavior that is rewarded (reinforced); and behavior *not* reinforced will, perhaps after an intervening period of time, occur less and less frequently.

A behavioral approach to the treatment of children with autism is also associated with certain program components. "Discrete trial" teaching is a core strategy in the Lovaas-UCLA model and most other behavioral programs for autistic children. What is meant by this term is direct instruction that focuses on one specific skill at a time, with repeated practice being provided on this task. Nelson's teacher was using discrete-trial teaching when she pulled him up from his chair three times and directed him to "sit down" each of these times. She will continue to repeat this process several times during the day over a period of perhaps weeks until Nelson has demonstrated consistently that he responds correctly to the phrase "sit down."

The term "applied behavior analysis" refers to a systematic process of observing and recording an individual's behavior, with the information collected being used to shape instruction and devise more effective intervention strategies. Applied behavior analysis provides the "technology" or tools for intervention. And yet in the end effectiveness is to a large extent determined by the knowledge, skills, and creativeness of the educators who collect and use the data to design individual educational treatment strategies.

Behavioral programs for young autistic children generally use a one-to-one teaching format all or most of the time. Thus, such programs are expensive, whether paid for by parents or by educational systems. In the long run they could prove to be economical by demonstrating a distinct advantage in enabling autistic students to enter mainstream educational programs later in childhood. At present, however, the assignment of one adult per child in publicly funded programs is rare, whether for preschoolers or for children five and over. What is seen much more frequently is classes with six to eight students, one teacher, and two teaching assistants.

In the preschool classes of the Douglass Developmental Disabilities Center at Rutgers University, the four members of the teaching staff are supplemented by a speech therapist who works in the classroom as well as by student teachers and psychology students. This arrangement allows a one-to-one format to be maintained. Other behavioral programs for young children with autism have to combine the one-to-one format with instruction for groups of two, but the value of individual instruction remains highly appreciated. The use of a one-to-one format has many advantages for teaching young children with limited understanding of language who spend large amounts of time in stereotyped behavior.

When the Lovaas behavioral model is working well, it goes something like this: as soon as autism is recognized an intensive (forty hours a week or close to it) one-to-one program is instituted in the home. When the child demonstrates that he or she can learn from observation, has some rudimentary communication skills, and does not exhibit tantrums, aggression, or self-injurious behavior with frequency—often six to twelve months after the program is instituted—he or she begins to attend a nursery school for typical children on a part-time basis, accompanied by a therapist from the in-home program. Initially the child may join the nursery school group for only one activity or thirty minutes a week, working his or her way up gradually to a whole morning or afternoon. After one to two years of therapy the child attends a nursery school program every day, still accompanied by a therapist who has been working with him in the home. Assistance from the therapist at school is carefully faded out, although the child continues to have one-to-one instructional sessions at home, on a somewhat reduced schedule. By the time the child is about six he or she begins attending either the first grade or a kindergarten class with children who are a year younger. Some special supports may be indicated, perhaps an individual teaching assistant part of the time or the provision of speech/language services, with the need for such support services decreasing over time.

Behavioral approaches, and Lovaas's program in particular, have been bombarded with criticism on two very different fronts—their successes and their shortcomings. After the 1987 publication of Lovaas's data that reported the recovery of 47 percent of the children in the Young Autism Project, some professionals attacked the outcome data. He excluded from his project those children who were very likely to have poor outcomes, a central criticism goes. To be admitted to the Young Autism Project, children had to be under forty months if they had no speech,

and under forty-six months if they had some speech; and the most retarded children were eliminated by IQ score cutoffs. Lovaas (1987) ac-
knowledged that some autistic children were excluded because of very
low mental ages; he stated that 15 percent of the population of young
autistic children would be excluded by this criterion. The project's
speech requirement for children forty to forty-six months of age undoubtedly excluded additional children. Even so, his achievement is impressive. The danger comes when parents of children who wouldn't
have been admitted to the Young Autism Project because they didn't
meet the admission criteria for age, speech, and/or mental age expect
their children to have an almost even chance of achieving normal functioning or something very close to it. They don't.

Professionals also attacked the use of the term "recovery." Having an
IQ at least in the average range and being able to progress in mainstream educational programs is not sufficient to demonstrate recovery,
they say. These criticisms may have some justification. Sandra Harris
found that the applied behavior analysis approach used in the preschool
program at the Douglass Developmental Disabilities Center was more
effective in improving IQ and language development than in improving
social behavior and relationships. Even so, what parent would not be
overjoyed if his or her autistic child met Lovaas's criteria for recovery?
Furthermore, in a later follow-up study of the nine children described
as having achieved normal functioning, Lovaas and his associates found
that only one of these children did not fall into the normal range on a
personality test and adaptive behavior scale; that particular student had
also been moved to a special education class (McEachin et al. 1993).

Lovaas makes a distinction between references to his outcomes as
cures or as recoveries. He states that he has never claimed to cure autism, that is, to have found and removed its cause, but he argues that
the use of the term "recovery" is justified for the children in his study
with the best outcomes. But the distinction between "cure" and "recovery" is subtle and easily lost. Personally, I think there would be less
danger of misleading parents and jumping to possibly incorrect conclusions if we could set aside the term "recovery."

Another criticism often directed against behavioral programs is that they produce rote or nonfunctional learning, that children learn to give certain responses during formal instructional sessions in the classroom but don't apply this learning in appropriate situations unless they are prompted to do so. Thus, a child may have learned to say "I want juice" during his work sessions, but doesn't use this language during lunch at school or at other times at home even if he likes and wants juice. In fact, such criticism was often justified in past years but is somewhat less often justified today. Good behavioral programs today include teaching in a variety of functional situations, for example, practicing use of language for requesting foods within the context of lunch, and practicing words about clothing in the context of a child putting on his hat and coat in preparation for going home. Such functional teaching does not replace formal instructional sessions using a discrete trial format; the two occur in tandem, complementing and supplementing each other, to promote generalization.

In a similar vein, programs derived from the Lovaas model have been criticized for focusing on reactive behavior, that is, teaching children to respond to adult directives and questions, to the detriment of spontaneity, initiative, and decision making. This criticism has considerable merit, although some behavioral programs have begun to modify their instructional planning to include opportunities for children to choose, decide, lead, and initiate. Still, this is an area in which there is much room for improvement.

Another source of concern about behavioral programs is their heavy reliance on nonprofessional "therapists," "trainers," or "teachers" (whichever term is used) who have little or no preparation for working with children other than the brief training they receive in a particular behavioral approach, and who provide almost all the direct instruction children receive. These therapists/trainers/teachers are generally college students or recent college graduates. Some of them consider that the model of behavioral intervention in which they have been trained is all they need to know because they believe that nothing else is of value in helping autistic children anyhow. Many of these young people are bright and dedicated, but when the specific techniques they have been taught don't seem to be effective for a particular child, they have no foundation to rely on in selecting and devising other types of teaching strategies. And they are often unaware of what they don't know about the development and education of young children. True, these teacher/therapists are supposed to be supervised by others with more skills and experience, but a Lovaas-type behavioral approach may also be the only approach that some of the supervising therapists (who may or may not be certified professionals) know themselves. "Do you know anything about Lovaas?" a young teacher/therapist asked me when I questioned her about why she did something a particular way (as if the Lovaas name was a sufficient explanation). "Yes, I do," I replied, "but that doesn't answer my question."

The most severe criticisms leveled against behavioral programs are criticisms of such approaches as they were implemented in the past. First, there is the association between behavioral programs and punishment. Yes, there was a time when Lovaas used electric shocks to try to eliminate certain types of behavior, and there was a long period when he used and advocated slaps to the buttocks for this purpose. Lovaas did include the use of a loud "No" and a slap on the thigh for undesirable behavior in his Young Autism Project (1987, 5); and Josh Greenfeld referred to a slap he witnessed when Lovaas was treating his son Noah: "Lovaas worked with Noah. . . . Usually he was gentle . . . but once when Noah reached out to take his reinforcer—or reward, the Frito— Lovaas slapped him down hard" (1972, 147). Many behavioral programs used "aversives" in their treatment during the 1970s.

Lovaas stopped administering electric shocks a long time ago, reportedly because the aggressive and self-injurious behavior they were designed to eliminate returned when the shock treatment was discontinued. He stopped using slaps more recently, and direct physical punishment has all but disappeared from behavioral treatment programs in the 1990s. Most parents of young autistic children won't tolerate their children being slapped, and a strong professional group, the Association for Persons with Severe Handicaps, has waged a strenuous battle against such practices. In a recent chapter of a book, Lovaas wrote: "In summary, we find that the use of aversives is unnecessary with most young children with whom we work" (1996, 242).

Still, there remains in some generally well regarded behavioral programs a sharpness or harshness that dismays many parents and professionals, including me. Restraint holds are used with young children in some school programs whenever the students exhibit aggression of any type or degree. This practice is built into a student's individualized education program with parental permission, and it may become a major intervention strategy. A teaching assistant uses a loud voice to address a five-year-old boy, with her face only a few inches from his. It is a strategy she has been taught for getting his attention. Stereotyped actions like hand flapping by a preschooler are reacted to with a loud "No." Such responses are derived, to some extent, from the considerable focus originally given by most behavioral programs to the elimination of undesirable behavior and from the blessing given by Ivar Lovaas to harsh intrusion and other kinds of tough treatment.

This harshness of response to children's behavior appears to be declining. I saw and heard a lot more hugging, kissing, tickling, swinging, praising, ignoring, and tolerating in most of the behavioral programs I visited during the past two years than I did sharpness. Furthermore, Lovaas appears to have given his stamp of approval to this shift and now seems to be urging his followers not to get locked into nonproductive routines. While he still sanctions physical restraint, Lovaas says that it shouldn't have to be used for more than a total of one or two hours ever. If you have to spend a great deal of time getting a child to sit in a chair, forget about sitting in chairs for a while, he says. If a child eats play dough, get rid of the play dough rather than spend a lot of time trying to eliminate that behavior. These messages have a very different tone than did his earlier ones. Furthermore, Lovaas has taken steps to reduce the trauma of the first treatment session by allowing the child to return to a parent for comforting frequently and by allowing the child to engage in ritualistic behavior for very short periods of time as a reward for doing what the adult directed.

And finally there are the children who stay in Lovaas-type programs for long periods of time as the gap between themselves and normally developing children grows wider and wider. What enthusiastic parents and professionals often forget is that slightly more than half of the children treated in the Lovaas program did not achieve normal functioning and that some made only modest progress although they stayed in the Young Autism Project treatment program for several years. One child was kept in treatment until his early teens, receiving more than 15,000 hours of therapy without acquiring much functional speech, and in the end his IQ had declined (Lovaas and Buch 1997, 82).

I again watched a videotape of five boys from the Lovaas Young Autism Project, three of whom were considered recovered, one considered to have made substantial progress, and one to have made only modest progress. Fourteen-year-old Chris, used as an example of modest progress, functions better than many autistic adolescents with severe mental retardation. Although he is in a class for retarded and autistic students, has an IQ of about 30, and uses signs because of his limited speech, we see him eating appropriately at the table with his mother and brother and shooting baskets in the family yard. No person and no approach produces good outcomes with all autistic children, even when intervention is started at a young age, as it was with Chris. Chris and his mother still had structured sessions focused on such tasks as naming objects from pictures. When Chris turned away during this session his mother told him sharply "Look." Whenever his face moved into a tic-like grimace she shouted "No faces!" For two years she had been teaching him to set their dining room table so that when he reached age twenty he might be able to work as a busboy. I wanted to tell this mother, very gently, that there are better ways to help her son to adulthood, that it was time to move on and probably had been for quite a while. How many times had she shouted "No faces!" at her son, I wondered.

A few weeks ago I visited a school for autistic children that uses a Lovaas approach and aims at recovery. How are the preschool children doing after a few years? I asked the director. We don't have the same recovery rate as Lovaas, she replied. A couple of our former preschoolers are now in inclusion programs, she told me, but for most of our preschoolers, placement in a less restrictive special education class is a more realistic goal. The children who make very modest gains stay here.

The Young Autism Project of Bancroft Rehabilitation Services in Haddonfield, New Jersey is one of the replication sites being operated in collaboration with Ivar Lovaas. The information booklet disseminated by that program in 1996 sounded a more modest note than did the 1987 and 1993 reports by Lovaas and his associates. The term "recovery" did not appear. The booklet announced that the goal of the program was the enhancement of intellectual, academic, social, and emotional behavior so that the child could take better advantage of socializing opportunities and require less long-term professional intervention. Bancroft also made no claims about helping children who had both autism and severe mental retardation. Children with mild to moderate retardation were the focus of the program, the information booklet stated clearly.

Most special education programs other than those based on the Lovaas model rely heavily on group instruction, and this factor may seriously reduce their effectiveness with children who have not yet broken the language code and still perceive the communications of others as a stream of meaningless sounds. Some time ago I observed a class for five-to seven-year-old autistic children in a public school. The teacher was a dedicated person who spent a good deal of time planning and preparing materials. She would have been an excellent teacher for typical or mildly disabled children in a pre-kindergarten class, but I doubt that her instructional efforts had much effect on all but one student in that class. Virtually all instruction was delivered to the group. The one child who had some receptive and expressive language, who could imitate and follow directions, seemed to be benefiting to some extent. He knew when the teachers were singing about him. He could retrieve the word card with his name on it when asked to do so. He could move his hands round and round like the wheels on a bus when a song about that was sung, and could hold up his fingers to match the words of another action song. The other children did not respond at all, apparently absorbed in their own worlds. From time to time an assistant teacher would guide a child's passive hands in motions matching the words of a song, or would point to an item of the child's clothing, but there was no indication that the child understood what anything meant. I watched this happen also in several preschool special education programs where group instruction was the primary format. In spite of the hard work of conscientious teachers, precious learning time was being wasted.

TEACCH, which stands for Treatment and Education of Autistic and Related Communication-Handicapped Children, is a statewide comprehensive intervention system that provides a variety of services to autistic individuals and their families across all age periods. Since 1972 the system has operated out of the department of psychiatry of the University of North Carolina, Chapel Hill, with state funding. It has an extensive training program for professionals and is also in use in other areas of the country as well as other parts of the world. Furthermore, Eric Schopler, the long-term (recently retired) director of the TEACCH system, has been a very influential figure in the autism field for many years.

The primary educational goal of TEACCH is to increase the student's level of skill. Recovery is not a term used in this system. While the Lovaas program is based on the premise that the child must overcome his autistic characteristics so as to adapt to the world around him, in TEACCH the child is provided with an environment designed to accommodate the characteristics of autistic children.

A TEACCH classroom makes use of many visual organizers or cues because visual processing is a strength of so many autistic children. Areas for special activities have clear boundaries. There are picture or picture-word schedules for individual children and for the class. Individual work systems are organized to maximize independent functioning and capitalize on the child's affinity for routines. Spontaneous functional communication is the language goal of TEACCH, and alternative modes of communication such as pictures, manual signs, and written words are used when speech is particularly difficult for the child. Such strategies neutralize or deemphasize deficits common in children with autism and minimize behavioral problems. While the TEACCH model uses individual instruction for some new skills, group instruction is a major format.

So, parents may ask, what's the bottom line? How effective is a TEACCH approach? This is not an easy question to answer. Unlike the Lovaas Young Autism Project, which served a small and select group of autistic children, TEACCH is open to all autistic children in the state of North Carolina and also serves students with communication problems who are not autistic. In addition, the TEACCH model is implemented in different settings such as mainstream classrooms and special classes. Over the years TEACCH has used a variety of measures to evaluate its effectiveness, including parent reports and rate of institutionalization. This latter measure was appropriate in the 1970s when the TEACCH model began; today, in the face of over fifteen years of deinstitutionalization, it is no longer a relevant outcome variable. Another outcome measure is parent satisfaction. A survey conducted by TEACCH in the late 1970s found that most parents were very satisfied with the services provided to their children and families. But the outcome measures that parents want to know about today are indices of children's performance. Given the long number of years that TEACCH has been in operation, the influence that this model has had in the area of treatment, and the major role that Eric Schopler played as a critic of the outcome data presented by Lovaas, it is surprising that TEACCH has not pursued comprehensive studies of child performance outcomes.

The data that are available on children served by TEACCH come largely from studies focused on stability of IQ (e.g., Lord and Schopler 1989a, 1989b) rather than on the effects of treatment per se. Based on these studies, Lord and Schopler report that substantial increases in IQ are common among children first evaluated at ages three or four, with the largest change found among children who were nonverbal and had IQ scores in the 30–50 range. These three-year-olds gained a mean of 22–24 points by age seven, while the four-year-olds gained an average of 15–19 points by age nine. However, most of these children still had IQs in the range considered to indicate mental retardation (Lord and Schopler 1994, 102), and the increases found in IQ between earlier and later test results may reflect differences in the tests themselves as well as changes in the children (1989a). Moreover, while a substantial number of children had increases of 20 points or more in IQ, decreases of this magnitude were found with equal or greater frequency among children first assessed after age three.

When asked, at the 1995 conference of the Autism Society of America, how many autistic children treated in TEACCH recovered, Eric Schopler, its long-term director, replied: "We have had some children who have become dissociated with the label of autism and others who have gone on to college." This was not quite the kind of answer parents were looking for.

While TEACCH doesn't have the same kind of outcome data as the Young Autism Project, I thought again of Chris, the fourteen-year-old on the Lovaas videotape who had made only modest progress. Had Chris been in the TEACCH system, his mother wouldn't have spent two years teaching him to set a table. The TEACCH program helps students acquire functional work skills, and the TEACCH system has well developed supported work programs for people like Chris. It also has all kinds of family support services for people like Chris's mother, and Chris might have expanded his life experiences and skills in a TEACCH summer camp with other adolescents. A mother who was attending the ASA conference explained to me that she returned to North Carolina when her autistic son reached adulthood because the state in which she lived for several years did not provide the variety and quality of services to adults with autism that the TEACCH system did. Her son now had a job he loved, she told me, because of TEACCH, which found the job, trained him for it, and provided enough on-going supervision to ensure that he would not lose it.

One major difference in overall strategy separating Lovaas-type programs and TEACCH is the different values assigned by these approaches to accommodating the child's autistic characteristics or waging an all-out war against them. This is not a one-time decision. Decision points on this issue continue to present themselves throughout the child's educational treatment. I faced such decision points with Victor when he was my student. Victor was almost ten and had been receiving treatment for about five years when one such point arose.

The science unit the class had been pursuing for almost two weeks was the prediction, measurement, and reporting of weather. As the most academically able student in this class, Victor kept our daily weather records. Each morning when he entered the classroom he took my copy of the New York Times, *turned to its weather page, and recorded on the chalkboard both the previous day's weather report and the predicted weather for the current day. The class then used this information in a variety of ways. One morning on my way to work, I noted that my bus was about to leave as I reached the corner where I usually boarded after buying a newspaper. My choice was to buy the paper and miss the bus or forego the newspaper and catch the bus. I caught the bus.*

When Victor entered the classroom that morning expecting to find the New York Times *on my desk but didn't, he was extremely upset. I had been ready to suggest that he borrow the* Times *from the teacher next door (who had been prepared by me for this request), but the suggestion came too late. For the next three hours until lunchtime Victor cried and screamed. I had not adequately accommodated his autistic difficulty in coping with unexpected events and changes in routines. On the other hand, the normal world would not abide by Victor's need for sameness. If he was to live in this world, he would have to learn to adapt to its unpredictability. Teaching Victor (and other students) to do so became the next instructional unit for the class and Victor's individual curriculum unit for many weeks to come.*

We focused on the idea that there are multiple ways to accomplish the same goal, and we practiced doing this in different situations, starting with the weather unit. I set the following question before the class: Suppose I were to forget to bring the Times *one day next week. How else could you get information about the weather? No one responded. I can think of one way, I said. Who else in the school has the* New York Times? *With this prompt Victor caught on, and in the next few days we borrowed the* Times *and other newspapers from various staff members. My next question to the class: Suppose one day no one had a newspaper? How else could we get a weather report? This time the prompt was not as useful, but we spent the next few days listening for the weather report on the radio, using the telephone to get the weather report, and going outside with a thermometer to record the temperature ourselves. Victor's homework was to listen to the weather report during the evening news. To make sure that Victor could make use of what we had been doing, I set one more question before him: Suppose I come in tomor-*

row without the Times. *What would you do for your morning weather re-cord? Victor went down the list of all the possible alternatives he could try. The next morning I "forgot" to bring the newspaper and Victor coped beauti-fully.*

From that point on, each time Victor appeared to be falling into an unvarying routine, we went back to our study of alternative means for reaching a particular goal. Had I continued to accommodate Victor's need for inflexible routines, he probably would have continued to have great difficulty coping in mainstream settings. Had I just insisted that he adjust, Victor's behavior might have deteriorated significantly. This balance between accommodation to autistic needs and adaptation to the expectations and demands of mainstream society must be handled with great care.

More than twenty years ago a mother faced this same decision about accommodating to or battling against autistic characteristics and wound up using both strategies in her successful struggle to help her son be-come more like his typically developing peers. Accommodation took the form of removal of all breakable or throwable objects and furniture from the home to reduce his violent behavior, but she fought against her son's insistence on sameness by systematically changing the arrange-ment of the remaining furniture and household routines, not allowing her son's protests and tantrums to deter her. To deal with her son's re-fusal to wear clothes, this mother purchased the few clothing items that appeared to attract him, and he began wearing one item continuously until he entered kindergarten and accepted the idea that he had to dress for school (Gajzago and Prior 1974).

The Delaware Autistic Program combines strategies from several mod-els, but the core of its approach with young children who enter without speech is a system called PECS. PECS stands for the Picture Exchange Communication System, a language training system that the Delaware program developed, field tested, and implemented. PECS has been gain-ing attention as a bridge to speech for young children with autism. Many autistic children have good visual skills but great difficulty in processing and producing speech. Thus, both manual communication and picture or picture-word systems of communication had been introduced when young children made very little progress in acquiring and using speech functionally. Manual communication or sign language has limited utility outside the deaf culture, and in actuality most autistic children acquire only a handful of signs—not enough to communicate effectively in most situations. Lack of an effective communication system is associated with increased tantrums, aggression, and even self-injury.

The Delaware Autistic Program doesn't wait until children in its programs have failed to respond to instruction. Its first language goal with the 80 percent of autistic children who enter its preschool programs without functional speech is to encourage the child to initiate communication, and to do so within the contexts of social activities and play. (This starting point differs markedly from the Lovaas program, which focuses initially on the production of speech sounds and word approximations along with the recognition of object names.) The child is taught to request desired items and activities by handing the adult a card with the picture of the item or activity on it. When the child does so, he is immediately rewarded by being given that item or allowed to engage in that activity. Some parents worry that the introduction of any communication system other than speech will interfere with the acquisition of speech. Not so, says Andrew Bondy, administrator of the Delaware Autism Program and one of the authors of PECS. Of the twenty preschoolers started on PECS during the 1987–92 period who stayed in the Delaware Autism Program for more than two years, fourteen (70 percent) use speech alone for communication, while another three (15 percent) use a combination of speech and PECS; only three children failed to acquire functional speech (Bondy and Frost 1994). Furthermore, many children begin to be able to use PECS on the first day it is introduced, thus eliminating another long period of time when they continue to lack any effective means of communication.

The most dramatic movement in special education in the late 1980s and early 1990s was the movement toward inclusion of students with severe

disabilities in the mainstream of education. The movement was bolstered by the provision in federal education law that students with disabilities should be educated in the least restrictive environment appropriate to their educational needs. This clause was used in the 1980s to
support the movement of students from special schools to regular neighborhood schools, and to limit the number of special education students
with mild to moderate disabilities placed in special classes. It wasn't
until the late 1980s that the inclusion movement began to attract significant numbers of parents of children with severe disabilities, and school
systems, prodded by the federal government, began to provide opportunities for such children to be included in the mainstream of education.

Why would the parent of a student with a severe disability want that
child to be in a class with typical children? For several reasons, including the fact that normally developing children can be excellent role models and teachers. A child who can learn by observing other children can
learn many desirable ways of acting and doing things from typical
peers. Is this really relevant to the education of autistic children, readers
may wonder. It certainly is for at least some, and inclusion matches the
dreams of parents of autistic children. They want their children in kindergarten, feeding the dolls, building bridges, painting pictures, sharing
and trading trucks with other children, and participating in "show and
tell"; not sitting in classrooms where the silence is punctuated by the
loud voices of teachers and the screaming of children, where the curriculum may revolve around "point to red," "put with same," "touch circle,"
and where children say nothing to one another.

Parents see the richness of programs for typical children and they
want some of that for their own autistic children. The critical questions
are: When can this richness benefit an autistic child, and when will it be
largely overwhelming confusion? How can we transform the richness
of what an autistic child may experience as a confusing maze into a
situation that expands the child's experiences, boundaries, and adaptive
capacities? Physical proximity to typically developing children does not
ensure that this will occur, and mainstream teachers do not find it easy
to support these goals. It's easier when the child comes with some skills
in communication and play, and there's an adult who knows him well

to help with the tough times. When this is not the case, it may take an inordinate amount of determination, dedication, and skill to make this experience beneficial for the autistic child.

A mother faced a dilemma. She was undecided about the best educational course for one of her children. Both of them were in a school program for autistic children that used a behavioral approach with one-to-one instruction. She felt very good about the progress of one child there, the one who had initially been less connected and responsive; but she wasn't sure about the benefits for her other child, who had always been more social and had shown few stereotyped behaviors before entering this program. Now her daughter had more of such behaviors. Was she imitating the other children, the mother wondered; and if so, shouldn't she be in a program where children were doing things that would be helpful to her? Should she be moved to an early childhood special education program with children who were not autistic so that she could observe other children who communicated and played together? Would her daughter do better in a typical preschool class with a one-to-one assistant teacher and speech/language therapy? Given her daughter's continuing difficulty in understanding speech, how much would she get out of the group instruction dominant in these programs? Many parents face such a decision, and there is no one answer that is always "correct."

The LEAP program (Learning Experiences . . . An Alternative Program for Preschoolers and Parents), located in Pittsburgh, Pennsylvania, began in 1982 as a federally funded model for the integration of autistic and typical children. The integrated preschool now has three classrooms, each with ten typically developing children and three children with autism. The children, ages three to five, are at the preschool three hours a day. A skills training program and support group meetings are offered to parents.

Activities specifically designed to facilitate language, social interactions, and adaptive behavior in the students with autism supplement the program's developmentally based early childhood curriculum. A variety of strategies are used to accomplish the program's objectives, including naturalistic teaching tactics like incidental teaching and play, direct instruction with reinforcement, peer modeling, and use of dramatic play teaching scripts. One strategy designed particularly well by this program is peer mediated learning. This involved training typical students to use facilitative strategies in interaction with their autistic classmates across a variety of situations, most notably play episodes in which two or three typical students are paired with an autistic classmate.

Research during the first twelve years of LEAP's operation showed that after two years in the program children generally showed a significant reduction in autistic symptoms and marked improvement on measures of intellectual development and language. Of the children with autism or PDD/NOS who spent two years in the program, twenty-four out of fifty-one are enrolled in regular education classes; some of these children had been enrolled in neighborhood kindergartens without any reference to their prior diagnosis (Strain et al. 1996).

LEAP is an exceptionally well designed program directed by highly skilled professionals. It combines naturalistic approaches with creative strategies for systematic teaching. Its outcomes are not likely to be duplicated by other programs with less carefully developed and researched instructional programs. Nor are its achievements likely to be matched by programs with less favorable structural supports such as class size and ratios of typical children to children with autism. What LEAP has demonstrated is that a Lovaas model is not the only approach that can produce good outcomes with young autistic children, and that under certain conditions the integration of typical preschoolers and children with autism can be highly productive.

Both the Delaware Autism program and LEAP use a combination of intervention strategies. In the spring of 1996 Stanley Greenspan declared his openness to doing the same. At an advanced clinical seminar he talked to his audience about combining models, including his developmentally based therapeutic approach and a behavioral approach. We should move away from the idea that all children have to fit into our program, he told his listeners. We want to adapt the program to fit the child's needs. Maybe a strategy from another program can be harnessed for this purpose, he added. With some children a behavioral approach may be used to get some basic patterns like imitation going, and developmental intervention can be used to put the pieces together—to help children integrate what they are learning or have learned.

It may well be, as Greenspan implied, that while a Lovaas-type behavioral approach can jump-start imitation, word naming, and some other basic skills, a developmental approach better addresses the weak "central coherence," the fragmented thinking with focus on details apart from context that is often characteristic of children with autism. According to Greenspan, emotions are the glue that pulls together fragments of learning, and developmental/therapeutic approaches are better at eliciting or tapping into such affect.

Many families with ample financial resources, in fact, already use combinations of approaches. Catherine Maurice implemented a full Lovaas program with both her children, but they also received developmentally based speech/language therapy three times a week. Other children who attend preschool programs using a behavioral approach receive sensory integration therapy after school hours.

"We can teach her one new skill, or five, or ten. . . . But there are hundreds of such skills inherent in the condition of a normal eight-year-old" (Park 1982, 263). This mother's lament highlights another important dilemma in educating autistic children. Autistic children don't learn much in the natural course of childhood activities and don't generalize from one situation to another unless their instructional programs give them extensive practice in doing so. (Even with such practice generalization is not assured.) How then can we possibly teach an autistic child all he needs to know to behave normally and acquire age-appropriate skills? The answer is that we can't if we try to teach every skill individually. The combination of autistic children's difficulty in generalizing and teaching approaches that focus on a series of single skills accounts for some of the inappropriate behavior and misconceptions seen in older children and adolescents with autism. In working with Victor, I attempted to teach him behavioral principles that would be relevant in many situations. Robert and Lynn Koegel and Laura Schreibman of the University of California have attempted to deal with this problem by focusing on what they call "pivotal behaviors"—behaviors that are likely to affect wide areas of functioning. In doing so, they are incorporating into an applied behavior analysis framework some of the more naturalistic teaching techniques common in preschool programs that have a developmental framework.

Robert Koegel and Laura Schreibman were involved in running the Lovaas autism program at UCLA in the 1970s. Since then they, together with Lynn Koegel, have evolved their own "brand" of intervention. The Koegels, who direct the Autism Research Center at Santa Barbara, and Laura Schreibman, who is now based at the University of California at San Diego, focus on such pivotal behaviors as motivation, responding to multiple cues, and self-management (Koegel et al. 1994; Koegel and Koegel 1995).

In an April 1997 conference presentation Robert Koegel reported that his own thinking about intervention was challenged by the lack of happiness apparent in the children in (Lovaas-type) behavioral programs even when they were making progress. He wanted children to want to learn to communicate and interact. In the attempt to make this happen, different objectives and methods came to the fore. In a Lovaas model, motivational considerations are generally limited to the identification of good reinforcers for a particular child. In the newer model advocated by the Koegels, the focus on motivation as a pivotal behavior brings into the process the child's preference or choice of instructional materials (stimulus materials, in behavioral terms), as well as teaching in the context of play and functional activities, and the use of natural reinforcers. The young child who points to a toy car and then looks at his teacher would get the opportunity to play with the car rather than eat a bit of food or enjoy some tickling. Instead of teaching colors by presenting construction paper circles or triangles of different colors, the teacher might hold out a handful of M & Ms. If the child takes an orange one, the teacher would say: "Orange. Take orange. What color is this? Orange." When all the orange M & Ms are gone, the same procedure could be repeated with the next color the child chooses, and the procedure could also be carried out with other kinds of items like balls. The reinforcement for the child is getting to eat the M & M or play with the ball—natural reinforcement that is very different from giving a child a Frito when he names a red circle correctly. Fritos might be used, according to Robert Koegel, to teach a child to open his lunch box when it contains this treat.

Recently, I visited a preschool with a Lovaas-type behavioral program. One little girl would not stay with her teacher during the formal discrete-trial instructional period. She kept leaving her seat and wandering around the room, listless, not appearing interested in anything in particular. "What's wrong with her today?" one of the other teachers asked. "She has no motivation," replied the girl's teacher. "All the [potato] chips are gone." Had Robert Koegel been there, he might well have commented: That's how we operated in the old days, and that's what needed to be changed.

In Koegel's newer approach the child has choice and more control. If a child is grumbling because he doesn't want to do something, he is told, "If you don't want to do it, say so." And if the child does this, he can change activities; again natural reinforcement. Much disruptive behavior disappears in this approach.

Responding to multiple cues is important because autistic children may identify a complex object or situation on the basis of only one or two marginal cues. Victor, for example, did not recognize the psychologist at the treatment center when she came into my classroom one day without her cane. Although she had tested him many times before, and he had always gone to her office willingly, on that day he refused to go with her, saying he didn't know her. Only after another student retrieved the psychologist's cane from her office did Victor recognize her. He then readily agreed to leave with her. Autistic children often have overselective attention.

Behavioral programs rely heavily on an adult's control of undesirable behavior by such means as extinction—the removal of reinforcers, including attention. Self-management as a pivotal behavior involves teaching the child skills such as the identification of appropriate behavior in different types of situations and the monitoring of his own behavior for such appropriateness. The process of self-monitoring shifts the locus of control to the child who then can function more independently.

Victor used to find it very hard to wait for my attention without becoming up-set, particularly when he wanted to ask me something about his work. But I had seven other students to work with in that class, and Victor's constant in-terruptions made it impossible for me to give the other students the help they needed. Since Victor could write, and he could understand why I couldn't al-ways respond to him immediately, we agreed to use the following procedure: when I was working with another child or children, Victor would write his questions in a small notebook to be kept on top of his desk specifically for this purpose. When I finished working with a particular child or group, I would check in with Victor and go over any questions in his book before I went on to work with another child or group.

Victor followed this procedure well and the situation improved immedi-ately. However, there were times when this strategy was inadequate, and Vic-tor still became upset at not having immediate access to me. Therefore, we worked on a back-up strategy. When using the question notebook was not enough, Victor was to change to a particularly soothing activity selected just for such times. Victor hit on the name of Upset Comforter for this activity. His first Upset Comforter was a United Nations flag coloring-book that indi-cated exactly what colors should be used on all parts of each flag. This exacti-tude fit well with Victor's need for certainty. With some prompting, Victor soon learned to recognize when it was time to get out his Upset Comforter. This was a strategy that Victor brought with him to his mainstream school and explained to his new teacher there.

In the 1987 *Handbook on Autism and Pervasive Developmental Disorders* Patricia Mirenda and Anne Donnellan suggested a useful direction for curriculum development: the marriage of different curricular ap-proaches, each contributing its particular area of strength. To a certain extent this is what is happening today in programs with a newer out-look. Along with systematic instruction, they incorporate "incidental teaching," which grows out of the child's interests and attempts at com-munication during the course of ongoing activities. They include recip-rocal play, in which a teacher and child take turns at blowing bubbles rather than have the teacher always do the bubble blowing and the child always be the reactor. They attend to the nature of antecedent variables, for example, types of activities, materials, and physical arrangements surrounding the instructional process, as well as to reinforcers. They focus more on how many object names a child uses in communicating during everyday activities than on how many pictures of objects a child can name. They stress proactive strategies and positive behavioral support rather than reactive and repressive responses to children's challenging behavior, focusing on building alternative behavioral skills rather than suppressing undesirable behavior. They work at developing children's skill and engagement in play. They accept the idea that sometimes the challenging behavior of autistic children is the child's only available means of communicating that he doesn't want to do something or needs to withdraw for a while from an overwhelming situation; and they recognize that sometimes the best way of "treating" this behavior is to give the child choices and respect them. Yet they do not sacrifice the particular strengths of applied behavior analysis—its ongoing assessment of the child's behavior and learning; its close linkage of assessment data and instructional planning; and its systematic instruction in basic processes.

A funny thing seems to be happening out there in the world of educational/therapeutic treatment of autistic children. Common elements are appearing in approaches that were considered very different, even antagonistic, as programs learn and borrow from each other. People seem more willing to acknowledge that maybe they haven't had all the right answers. The director of a school that describes its goal as recovery and its approach as applied behavioral analysis told me: Maybe it's time to think of a TEACCH model for some children who show few signs of movement toward recovery after a year or two. The more gentle and loving hand long espoused by programs based on a developmental approach seems to be creeping into programs derived from the Lovaas framework; and the principal theorist of developmental intervention, Stanley Greenspan, is talking about combining behavioral and developmental approaches to better fit the needs of some children.

What Lovaas does better than anyone else is document outcomes, both short-term and long-term. (He should soon have data from his replication sites.) Very few other programs carefully collect outcome data. While there are many justifications for this lack—it's time consuming and expensive to measure outcomes and follow-up on children, for example—this is information that parents feel they need in making decisions that may significantly affect their children's futures. It's one of the major reasons why parents are flocking to programs using Lovaas-based approaches. Parents who have options are no longer willing to take the word of a high-status professional that his or her approach works. Nor are they satisfied with research that only provides narrowly based short-term data. They are saying, "Show me. My child's whole future is at stake, and it's too precious to entrust to some professional's say-so. What data do you have to support your claim of effectiveness?" Program directors and researchers should heed this message. (Even the promising practices reported by the Koegels need to be examined within a broader context.)

Educational treatment of autistic children has come a long way but is still only moderately effective with many children. To a significant extent this result reflects the fact that education is not a cure or even the optimal treatment for the neurobiological differences that underlie the condition or conditions currently called "autism." To a lesser extent the modest result of educational treatment reflects poor implementation or a mismatch between children's needs and programs' strategies. Parents may very much want to implement thirty- to forty-hour weekly in-home programs for their two- or three-year-olds who have been diagnosed as autistic but can't because of other demands on their time combined with limited financial resources. Some school programs may be so "eclectic" that no specific instructional strategies are implemented with the intensity and consistency needed by autistic children. Many school systems are still not receptive to the movement of autistic children into inclusive settings along with the specialized supports and strategies they are likely to need. Yet this step is essential to the progress of a substantial number of children with autism toward fuller social development.

There is no room for complacency in the battle against autism. The tools we have to work with today are only effective when wielded with what Raun Kaufman, a young man who used to be called autistic, referred to as "passionate relentlessness."

7 Whatever Happened to Equal Opportunity?

Intensive one-to-one teaching for developmentally

disabled children starting at the age of 2

should be an entitlement.

(Interview with Ivar Lovaas 1994, 21)

All over the country in-home programs are springing up for two- to four-year-old children diagnosed as autistic. Most of these programs are derived from the Lovaas/UCLA Young Autism Project model. Parents of preschoolers, after hearing about the "47 percent recovery rate" in this project, began rejecting the preschool special education classes that school districts offered; or they accepted these programs initially but— when their children showed little or no obvious improvement after a few months—switched to the in-home Lovaas model. These parents were so determined not to allow anything to interfere with their children's progress toward recovery that they paid for the in-home services themselves initially and then fought for reimbursement later. Of course, only some families can gather the money to pay for an intensive in-home program when reimbursement is questionable and at best far down the road. Not families whose income is barely above the poverty level; not families of five living on the salary of a firefighter or a teacher,

119

no matter how much they want such treatment for their autistic child. Even for the upper-middle-income families of many lawyers and doctors the costs can be staggering, but these are the families who can and do stretch enough to undertake the costs of forty-hour-a-week in-home programs.

What are the costs? The UCLA Clinic for the Behavioral Treatment of Children offers training workshops to families to enable them to set up their own in-home programs based on the Lovaas model. The clinic recommends an initial two- to three-day workshop, with a follow-up workshop every three or four months. The fees charged by the UCLA clinic in 1996 were $1,700 plus airfare, ground transportation, hotel, and $30 per diem for two days; $2,300 plus the other charges for three days. To these workshop charges, and additional fees for telephone or videotape consultations parents may wish to use, add the cost of ongoing direct instruction. Lovaas recommends that families recruit a staff of at least three therapists, preferably undergraduate students, to implement the treatment program, as very few families can provide thirty to forty hours a week of instruction without some assistance. Another alternative suggested by Lovaas is that parents recruit and use volunteers to provide this instruction, with the family paying one person to supervise the whole program; $15,000 might cover that, he indicated. But only a few families manage to operate the program with unpaid volunteers, he remarks.

Bancroft Rehabilitation Services in New Jersey, a replication site for the Lovaas model, recommended the following training for parents planning to implement the Lovaas in-home program: an initial three-day training workshop ($1,500), with follow-up workshops of one or two days ($700 or $1,100) every six to ten weeks. Bancroft also offers two other follow-up services for parents—telephone consultations ($60 per hour) and videotape consultations at the same hourly rate. A panelist at the April 1995 Westchester conference on behavioral approaches to autism estimated the total cost of implementing the Lovaas in-home program as $3,500 to $4,000 a month, that is, $42,000 to $48,000 per year. One New York City father calculated his family's expenditures for his autistic son's first year of education as over $50,000, which included the in-home behavioral program, additional speech/language services, a part-time nursery school experience, and a variety of evaluations and consultations; other families in New York City have also identified one-year expenditures for their preschool child at $40,000 to $50,000.

But what about families whose annual income is less than $50,000, a category that includes a large segment of the American population, and parents who don't have extended family members who can give or lend them money for this purpose? What about their children's progress toward "recovery"? What about single-parent families where that parent must work and try to juggle the coordination and monitoring of an in-home program as well as its cost? The Lovaas/UCLA in-home model is easiest to implement and works best when the family is intact and generously endowed with several kinds of resources: money, intelligence, emotional resilience, and a good natural support system made up of friends, neighbors, and relatives.

A letter from a mother in the newsletter of the Autism Society of America raised the broad issue of differences in family resources and how children's futures are affected by them:

> As it says in the autism definition, "It has been found throughout the world in families of all racial, ethnic, and social backgrounds." We are one of those families, and though we adore our daughter, Merav, she spent almost eight years in the children's unit of the state hospital, in Austin, Texas. We just didn't have the funds, or the contacts, to get her into a private residential program of our choice when it became apparent that she, and us [sic], needed immediate help.
>
> Please give more thought to the struggles people like us face. We do the best we can under the circumstances. With little income . . . with no family within a 1,000 mile radius. . . . Our children are our life. Please . . . write something about people like us who make less than $40,000 a year, have a seven-year-old car, and still rent because we can't afford to buy a house. We love our children, we just can't afford the P.R. man. (Schloss 1995, 5; reprinted with permission of the Autism Society of America)

School districts have little experience at supporting in-home programs and are much more comfortable with center-based programs. Yet in-home programs for young children have a long history. They began expanding in the late 1960s and early 1970s, along with a focus on the prevention of school problems in children then labeled "disadvantaged," many of whom had IQ scores in the borderline or mildly retarded range. Paraprofessionals were the direct-care workers in some of these programs. Thus, the Lovaas model was hardly the earliest in-home model or the first to use noncertified personnel to provide direct services. But school districts rarely took part in these in-home programs, which drew support from a combination of sources other than state and local public education funds. The only experience that most school districts had with in-home programs was through the home instruction services they provided to school-age children with physical or health impairments. In the 1970s such services came to be identified as highly restrictive and were largely phased out. In-home programs for preschool children as an alternative to special education classes were not within the experience base of most public school systems until very recently, when itinerant teacher models became more common.

School systems that cannot provide appropriate education for school-age children with disabilities must pay for such educational services to be provided elsewhere. This was not always the case. Until the passage of the Education for All Handicapped Children Act of 1975, children with severe disabilities like autism were often excluded from public education. With very few nonpublic options open to them, many of these children wound up without any educational services. The 1975 law dramatically changed that situation by introducing the concept of public responsibility for the education of *all* children, no matter how severe their disabilities. All children of school age were to receive a free and appropriate public education. Following the passage of this law, large school districts moved to develop programs for autistic children of school age, while small school districts provided such services through intermediate or county programs. A great inequity had been redressed, and a severe service gap had been filled.

Until December 1986 federal law did not require states to provide services to preschool children with disabilities unless they provided such services to nondisabled preschool children, although states were given financial incentives to do so. Therefore, parents had no legal foundation from which to seek funding for in-home programs. The situation changed with the passage of the 1986 Amendments to the Education of the Handicapped Act, which required states to provide a free and appropriate education to children with handicaps aged three to five. Furthermore, a new section of this education law, Part H, introduced the idea of services to infants and toddlers from birth to age three and encouraged states to provide such early intervention services. By September 1994 all states had established systems of early intervention services. The legal foundation needed to allow parents to fight for the programs they wanted for their infants, toddlers, and preschoolers had been put into place. Moreover, while most preschool programs are provided at agency sites, the home is the most common setting for the delivery of early intervention services to children below age three.

Today a new inequity faces us. It is not about the right to service; that battle has been won, at least for parents who know how to find out what services their child is entitled to and how to go about getting them. Many parents of infants, toddlers, and preschoolers—young, inexperienced, with limited educational backgrounds and poor natural support systems—may not recognize that something is going wrong in their child's development, that their child should be evaluated without delay, and that their child is entitled to such an evaluation without any cost to them. Federal special education law provides that each state must ensure that all children with disabilities who are in need of special education services are identified and evaluated. While a comprehensive child-find system is mandated, a substantial number of children of parents who are very poor are still not identified and evaluated until age four or five. Given what we know about the importance of early intervention for children with autism and other pervasive developmental disorders, this is a situation in need of significant improvement.

Today the primary battle in progress is about the right to appropriate services, that is, about what is appropriate and who decides this. Put simply, when parents believe that the programs offered by school systems do not meet their children's educational needs, the parents with ample financial resources are the ones most likely to be able to obtain alternative programs at public expense. Let's look at an example of how this might happen by returning to Westchester, where the conference featuring Ivar Lovaas was held in April 1995. That conference was part of a fund-raising effort by a parent organization whose goal was to develop a school for autistic children that would use the Lovaas framework. It had taken the parents about two years to reach that point. In 1993 several couples with young autistic children came together to pool their resources with the objective of obtaining public funding for in-home programs using an applied behavior analysis approach. Some of these parents were already implementing and paying for such programs, sometimes after trying and then rejecting special education preschool programs recommended by their local school districts. These parents had already sought reimbursement from their health insurance companies but had not been successful for a combination of reasons. Now their target was the county of Westchester, whose approval was essential if in-home programs were to become an approved educational option for their children.

These parents knew what they were doing; some had legal backgrounds. They organized committees to work on different aspects of their advocacy. They lobbied politicians and met with the relevant educational decision makers at state and local levels. They threatened lawsuits. The county began to show some interest and called a meeting for parents and directors of state-approved preschool programs. One agency agreed to sponsor the in-home programs. Its plan was approved by the county, and public funding was provided. The agency added to its staff the "therapists" parents were already using, paying them as paraprofessionals for a total of thirty-eight hours a week per child. Two hours a week of supervision was provided by a trained behavioral specialist with certification in special education. Having achieved the goal of publicly supported in-home Lovaas-type programs for their preschoolers, the parent organization moved on to other objectives, with establishment of a school for children who needed to continue to receive intensive services after age five being at the forefront.

The Westchester story is a good story. It shows public education at its best—recognizing and supporting an option that might meet the needs of some autistic children better than any of the existing alternatives. A critical question that can not be ignored is whether other citizens, less affluent and less knowledgeable about how to influence public systems, are obtaining or could obtain equal consideration and a similar expansion of educational options for their children.

Let's look at a second group of parents who wanted exactly what the Westchester parents had obtained for their children. This second group was not based in an affluent suburban area. It was based in Staten Island and drew families from at least three other boroughs of New York City. In January 1995 the first meeting of this just revived parent organization, the Autism Advocacy and Outreach Group (AAOG), attracted close to a hundred parents and others. The first part of the meeting was spent in airing complaints and giving voice to frustrations: Parents had to scrape together every penny they had to pay for a few hours a week of in-home behavioral services, and they knew that this was insufficient; there weren't enough schools in New York City using this approach, and the public school system was not receptive to their pleas for such services. A determination to fight for what they considered their children's only hope was obvious. Then came a presentation by one of the mothers from the Westchester parent organization on the strategies used by that group to achieve the services they sought. The remainder of the meeting was devoted to questions about implementation of these strategies.

An attorney from the New York Lawyers for the Public Interest was the speaker at the second AAOG meeting. This nonprofit law office had been designated as the protection and advocacy agency for people with developmental disabilities in New York City. (Under federal developmental disabilities laws dating back to the 1970s, each state had to have in operation a system to protect and advocate for the rights of persons with developmental disabilities.) This agency had agreed to work with the parents in AAOG to help them obtain appropriate services for their children. As a starting point a letter had been sent to relevant persons within the public school system outlining the issues and objectives. Over the next few months meetings were held, some with school district representatives. A proposal for specific new services was invited and submitted, but no new programs were initiated by the board of education either for preschool children or young school age children. Some nonpublic agencies providing special education services in New York City were, however, beginning to listen to parents, and in September 1995 a couple of behavioral programs for preschool children were started. But these were center-based programs—the quest for publicly funded, intensive, Lovaas-type in-home programs for preschoolers was not successful. In the meantime, movement through legal pathways was slow (though a few individual cases were resolved), and parents became increasingly discouraged about being able to obtain the intensity of services the Westchester families had in time to help their own children.

In Westchester, as 1996 approached the parent organization moved closer to opening its new behavioral school for autistic children of five and over. In New York City parents who believed that public school classes for autistic students aged five, six, or seven held no hope for their own children continued to hire private advocates to help them get approval for nonpublic school placements. That is, if they could afford the fees that such private advocates charged. And even then, the "victory" was sometimes of limited value because the number of nonpublic schools serving autistic children with the kind of program that the parents sought was very small, and some had waiting lists.

What is happening in other parts of the country about the provision of in-home options for preschool children? Let's look at some recent legal decisions relevant to this question. A synthesis of such cases has been prepared by Iowa Protection and Advocacy Services, Inc. (Swanson and Sytsma 1995). In three of the cases parents were seeking public funding for the actual Lovaas/UCLA clinic program. In two other cases parents were seeking public funding for in-home Lovaas-type programs in other states. In the sixth case the parents sought funding for placement in a private school with a behavioral approach rather than in a district special education preschool program where a "blended" approach was used. Of these six cases judicial decisions favored the parents in four instances and the school district in one, with the remaining decision being mixed.

The judgment favoring the school district came in the earliest of the six cases (*G. F. v East Hanover Board of Education*, 1989) and the only case in which parents sought funding for placement in a private school. In that case, the administrative law judge ruled that the district's proposed program met both federal and New Jersey state definitions of appropriate as "sufficient to confer some educational benefit" (79). A 1982 Supreme Court decision (*Board of Education v Rowley*) had clearly indicated that "appropriate" does not mean optimal benefit or maximum possible benefit, although a 1988 decision by the Third Circuit court clarified this further by indicating that "appropriate" implied benefit that was meaningful, not trivial or minimal. The Supreme Court decision also indicated that when there are competing methodologies at issue, the professional judgment of the educational agency should prevail.

In the mixed judgment case (*In re Calaveras Unified School District*, 1994), the original program offered by the California school district was found deficient, but the revised individualized education program was found appropriate. Therefore, reimbursement was ordered for the period during which the proposed program was not appropriate, but funding was denied from the time that an appropriate individualized education program was offered. The revised program offered by the school district included a one-to-one teacher aide at school, a behavior management program, structured speech/language services, parent training, participation with nondisabled students in a Head Start class at the same site, and twenty hours a week of individual instruction in the home delivered by a teaching aide.

In the four cases supporting the parents, the programs offered by the school districts were found deficient in a variety of significant ways, while the in-home programs were found to be appropriate. Thus, the school districts were ordered to reimburse the parents for assorted costs associated with delivery of the in-home programs. In one of the cases (*M. A. v Voorhees Board of Education*, 1994) the school district was found to have taken a careless approach to the education of the child when the needs of this child dictated a systematic, intensive instructional program.

The families in these cases had the financial resources to pay for in-home programs and hire attorneys to fight for reimbursement later. In fact, the families in two of these cases rented apartments near the UCLA clinic that the child attended and periodically flew back to their homes in San Diego. Clearly, such families have open to them options not generally available to families of more modest means. However, some state protection and advocacy agencies are now working to assist families prospectively rather than through reimbursement for funds already spent. To the extent that such efforts succeed, they will significantly reduce the present state of inequity of educational options based on financial resources.

An October 1995 letter from Mary Jane White accompanied the synthesis of cases compiled by Iowa Protection and Advocacy Services. Mary Jane White reported that her family was the second Lovaas case handled by Iowa Protection and Advocacy Services. Her initial contact with this agency took place in December 1994. By October 1995 sixteen other families known to this agency were receiving full or partial funding for Lovaas-type in-home programs from school districts in Iowa, and other families were in the process of negotiating such funding, assisted either directly or indirectly by the work of the Iowa protection and advocacy agency.

All the activities described above related to the educational treatment of children of three years or over, but recently there has been an explosion in the number of two-year-olds being identified as PDD/NOS. Two-year-olds are not considered part of the educational system in all states as are three- and four-year-old preschoolers. The Individuals with Disabilities Education Act (IDEA), which is the current name for the federal education law on children with disabilities, treats children from birth through age two differently than children three and over. It gives each state the right to choose the lead state agency for the provision of comprehensive, interagency services to infants and toddlers; only about a third of the states chose education, with another third choosing health, and most of the remainder choosing the state developmental disabilities agency. Furthermore, while IDEA guarantees that services to children ages three and older will be free of cost to the parent, there is no such guarantee for children under age three. States were given the right to establish sliding-fee scales for family payment if this practice was consistent with state law, although states cannot deny services because of a family's inability to pay or charge any family for evaluations. Payment for early intervention services to children below age three must be sought from such sources as private health insurance and Medicaid before funds provided through Part H of IDEA may be used, unless this causes a delay in the provision of timely services to the child.

The need to seek private insurance funding for early intervention services is a source of concern to many families, particularly in relation to annual or lifetime maximums on coverage. In order to deal with this real problem, some states have incorporated protections into state law to cover this situation. New York State, for example, prohibits insurers from charging any benefits paid for early intervention services against such caps.

In-home services are the most common form of service delivery for infants and toddlers under IDEA. Thus, one of the objections of some school systems to in-home programs for preschoolers is moot in relation to toddlers. (In addition, behavioral programs often rely heavily on paraprofessionals.) On the other hand, the intensity of services provided to infants and toddlers has generally been low. In some states the norm was two hours a week until very recently, and children with autism or PDD/NOS who needed more hours of dedicated interaction and instruction could get them only if their parents could pay for or provide the additional services themselves.

Parents have approached the problem of obtaining funded intensive services for their toddlers in two main ways: through advocacy and through legal channels, with their targets being health insurance companies and Part H (infant/toddler) services under IDEA. There are multiple roadblocks to obtaining reimbursement for in-home programs through health insurance. Aside from the broad movement to cut medical costs by limiting the amount and types of services covered, some health insurers still try to treat autism as a form of mental disorder that is subject to strict coverage ceilings, while other plans specifically exclude treatment of autism and other developmental disorders. Difficulties also derive from the fact that services are often delivered by persons who are not considered health care professionals. Thus, a health plan that may provide some coverage for services delivered by a licensed speech/language therapist is not likely to cover any of the cost of direct services by the noncertified or licensed educational therapists who deliver most of the direct services for in-home programs. At every conference on autism numerous parents bring up this problem of health insurance companies that fail to provide coverage or adequate coverage for autism treatment, calling the problem to the attention of the psychiatrists and other physicians present. Their answers are never satisfying to parents. Yet on the basis that autism is a neurological rather than a psychological disorder, some parents have succeeded in obtaining reimbursement for their expenses. One case that established a legal precedent for such reimbursement is *Kunin v Benefit Trust Life Insurance Company.* In 1990 the U.S. Court of Appeals for the Ninth Circuit affirmed a decision of a U.S. District Court in California that autism is not a form of mental illness and that benefits could not be limited on such grounds.

Parents are increasingly channeling their energies into fighting for services under the infant/toddler provisions of IDEA. In early 1995 I spoke to an early intervention service coordinator in New York. Most infants and toddlers were receiving two hours a week of services, she told me, but some parents of two-year-olds with diagnoses of autism or PDD/NOS had pressed hard for more and were now getting up to eight hours of service. A year later I spoke to this coordinator again. Five or six lawsuits initiated by parents were now pending in New York City, she reported. The issue was intensity of services, that is, number of hours provided. The service limits had already been pushed upward, with the maximum being sixteen hours a week of in-home services, and with a precedent established for children to receive combinations of center-based and in-home services that together exceeded twenty hours. What the parents who had filed lawsuits wanted was reimbursement for forty-hour-a-week in-home programs. Two of the cases were on appeal. In one, the administrative law judge had ruled against the parents. In the other, the judgment had favored the parents. To some extent the activities of parents with greater financial resources who paid for the in-home programs of their toddlers and then fought for reimbursement benefited parents with more limited financial resources as well. The legal actions of the former parents led to an expansion of service hours for other parents and stimulated the initiation of new programs for toddlers.

While parents in New York City were fighting for intensive early-intervention services for their two-year-olds, so too were parents in Westchester. The success of parent efforts in gaining intensive services for preschoolers did not carry over to toddlers. In New York State services to preschoolers are the jurisdiction of the New York State Education Department, while services to infants and toddlers are under the direction of the New York State Department of Health. Thus, there was a different bureaucracy to deal with and a new battle to be waged.

Some parents, being unable to afford thousands of dollars each year to supplement the meager amount of service time provided through early intervention programs, have used creative means, born of determination, to arrange for more hours of educational treatment. In Sacramento, California a group of parents formed an organization they named Families for Early Autism Treatment (FEAT), devoted to delivering cost-effective in-home intervention based on the Lovaas/UCLA model (Huff 1996). FEAT implemented a variety of fund-raising activities; arranged for sharing training and the costs associated with it; recruited volunteers and students who would receive college credits for their work; arranged for the sharing of toys and instructional materials; and provided a support network for parents managing in-home programs.

The use of students who work for college credit, while a much sought-after way to reduce the cost of in-home programs, is often not satisfactory in practice because of student absence during college intersessions, their high turnover rate, liability concerns, and the reluctance of many colleges to provide internship credit for in-home programs. At the University of California, Irvine these constraints were greatly reduced by the establishment of a formal internship program for in-home programs. A private foundation was created that bought liability insurance; listings were placed in campus internship directories to recruit more students; a centralized computer database of parents and students was created to assist in matching schedules; and once-a-month lectures on various aspects of autism by professionals with different points of view or information to contribute were made mandatory for student interns. Several other nearby colleges and hundreds of students have participated in this program (Kenneth Pomeranz, personal communication, November 26, 1996).

A strategy sometimes used by parents, both for financial reasons and because they believe their children have reached a point where they can benefit from small group instruction under carefully planned circumstances, is to combine a preschool special education experience with an in-home behavioral program of reduced hours. The Irvine, California school district has collaborated with parents to design and support such a combined program (Kenneth Pomeranz, personal communication, November 26, 1996). The school district pays a senior therapist for two hours a week to oversee the in-home program and the integration of home and school programs. The senior therapist is often the person the parent had already been using to supervise the in-home program. The school district also pays for a five-to-six hour-a-week "bridge therapist" who works directly with the child to ensure the smooth implementation of the school and home programs. For other children, who are included full-time in preschool programs for typically developing children, the school district provides a "shadow." A "shadow" might best be thought of in educational terminology as an assistant teacher assigned to work with an individual special-needs child in an inclusive setting. Such supported inclusion helps children with autism acquire the skills they need to function well in the educational mainstream. The collaboration between the Irvine school district and parents offers a welcome contrast to the contentious relationships and legal maneuvering that characterize relationships between parents and the educational establishment in many other parts of the country.

A year has passed since I attended the Westchester conference on behavioral intervention in autism. In a few days a 1996 version of that conference—same sponsoring organization, same subject, same place, and some of the same speakers—will take place. I am looking at the conference brochure, trying to decide whether to go. Instead, I pick up the telephone and call the African-American mother from Brooklyn whom I met at the conference last year. It's been several months since I tried to reach her, and her son must be six by now, I realize. This time I do reach her. None of the promises of help that were made at the conference last year have materialized except a parent outreach program. Her son is still in the same class in the same school, doing about the same. Now she feels a new need to push for something else. Individual speech/language services will no longer be provided to her son in the public school program he attends, this mother tells me. All such services will be delivered to groups of students in the classroom. She's trying to find a private advocate or attorney whom she can afford, to fight for her son's placement at a private school that uses a Lovaas-type behavioral model. The advocate she had called would not talk to her without a $600 payment up front. What this mother wants for her son is some kind of a life, some kind of a future in which he can be productive and will have satisfying experiences. She doesn't see him being helped toward that now.

And what of the parents from the Autism Advocacy and Outreach Group based in Staten Island who fought for Lovaas-type in-home programs for their toddlers and young preschoolers? Most of their children received considerably less than forty hours a week of in-home services, but many of these children found places in a private preschool serving autistic children that receives public funding and uses a Lovaas-type behavioral approach. Some of the children have made substantial progress, while others are still struggling with the basics of understanding and communicating. At the same time, the Westchester school founded by the parent group described earlier is open and thriving.

Undoubtedly, the service picture for young children with autism today is much brighter than it was in the past, but it is still not bright enough. The years before age six or seven are critical years for battling the debilitating aspects of autism. Services that are skimpy will not do, and a society that values equal opportunity cannot afford to tolerate inequities that may have lifelong consequences. The tenor of the times in the second half of the 1990s does not favor new entitlements, so I doubt very much that Lovaas's entitlement recommendation of intensive one-to-one teaching for two-year-olds (1994, 21; quoted at the beginning of this chapter) has any chance of being heeded. But steps do have to be taken—by states, counties, and local educational authorities, by parents individually and in organized groups, by disability advocacy organizations, and by educators—to ensure that economic factors do not deprive some autistic children and their families of the collaborators they need in the struggle to achieve a decent life.

8 Some Thoughts on Alternative Treatments and Other Intervention Controversies

Because most children with autism don't "recover" or achieve near-normal functioning, and because many children with autism struggle for years against formidable challenges to their understanding and happiness, parents and professionals continue to search for better answers. The search for a cure for autism is fifty years old. Detours and false starts mark the way, along with optimism and "miraculous cures" that turned out to be less than miraculous and less than a cure.

Perhaps the most damaging detour was the belief that autism was caused by parental behavior toward the child, particularly by the cold rejection of the mother. Leo Kanner, the child psychiatrist who first brought attention to the condition referred to as autism, inadvertently led the way into this detour. While Kanner believed that autism grew out of an innate inability to form relationships, he also referred to the "emotional frigidity in the typical autistic family" and to the "dramatically evident detachment, obsessiveness, and coldness that is almost a

135

universal feature of parents of autistic children" (Eisenberg and Kanner 1956, 561).

The view of autism as reflecting an inborn defect in relating did not fit the zeitgeist of the 1950s and most of the 1960s. That era was permeated by psychoanalytic perspectives on child dysfunction. If autistic children were cut off from and nonresponsive to the significant others in their lives, it was assumed that this resulted from something the child was deprived of, something parents should have done but didn't; or perhaps something parents shouldn't have done but did. The era of blaming parents for their child's autism was in full bloom.

What Kanner and other professionals did not consider was the process of reciprocal interaction—initiation and reinforcing response—that takes place between parents and their normally developing babies, and the effect on parents of having a nonresponsive child who is also difficult to understand and manage. What professionals also did not consider was that the parental behavior they were witnessing might have been the end result of a long period of uncertainty, doubt, and stress about their child's development. (Still another hypothesis posed recently in light of growing evidence of genetic involvement in autism is that some of the parents of autistic children seen by Kanner may themselves have been mildly autistic or had Asperger's syndrome.)

Given this view of autism as a form of emotional disturbance growing out of a lack of warm and loving care during the early years, psychodynamic treatment approaches dominated the 1950s and 1960s. Thus Virginia Axline in her 1964 book, *Dibs in Search of Self*, presented her young patient as being cured through play therapy. And Bruno Bettelheim, the most notorious blamer of parents, claimed cures of autistic children through psychodynamic milieu therapy after separating children from their families. Many of the claims made by Bettelheim have been vigorously disputed, and Axline's success in using play therapy with "Dibs" was rarely replicated with severely impaired autistic children. It was a parent-professional, Bernard Rimland, who in his 1964 book, *Infantile Autism*, presented the evidence against psychogenic interpretations of autism so compellingly that a death knell began to sound for these views. At the same time, the search for an organic cause of autism gained much needed vigor.

Good research is a time-devouring process. Small chunks of a problem are tackled one by one as hypotheses are generated and explored. As layers of information accumulate, researchers construct or modify theories to fit all the known pieces. The search for the organic or neurobiological underpinnings of autism has recently taken on new momentum. Bolstered by technological advances, research has begun to yield very promising clues. However, cures or even highly effective treatments for autism tied to its neurobiological origins still appear to be a long way off. In the meantime, parents of autistic children wait impatiently and look elsewhere, grasping at promising possibilities.

Today's promising possibilities, most with minimal supportive evidence from careful research, are the treatment alternatives to which parents with resources are flocking, and in which they invest not only their money but also their dreams. From a researcher's point of view these parents are investing in hypotheses or educated guesses. From the parents' point of view the results of thorough research may come too late for their own child. I asked a psychiatrist who is highly regarded and highly published in the area of autism what he thought of treatment with prednisone for children diagnosed with autism of late onset who had EEG patterns like those in Landau-Kleffner syndrome. "It's premature," he replied. In a sense he's right, particularly since these drugs can have perilous side effects; but to the parents of a child who has lost the ability to speak and to understand speech, and who appears less and less able to participate in the joys of childhood, the risk might be well worth taking.

Today's controversial alternative treatments may become the discarded guesses of tomorrow, but one or more of them may turn out to be an effective form of treatment for a substantial number of autistic children. In the meantime, using them involves a balancing act, with risks being weighed against potential benefits.

Bernard Rimland has devoted most of his adult life to identifying and tracking possible treatments for autism. In the process, working out of the Autism Research Institute in San Diego that he founded in 1967, he brought to the attention of parents and professionals most of the alternative treatments used today. He also personally championed several treatments whose efficacy he believed in but most other professionals didn't. Megavitamin therapy is an alternative treatment that Rimland has studied for over twenty years. He believes fervently in the value of vitamin B6 for a substantial proportion of the autistic population and advocates daily supplementation with B6 and magnesium, preferably through a megavitamin formulated for this purpose. What such treatment accomplishes in about 35 to 50 percent of autistic children, according to Rimland, is improvement in attention and learning, along with decreases in hyperactivity and irritability. Some recent research indicates that vitamin B6 may have a beneficial effect because it modulates the function of neurotransmitter enzymes. Abnormalities in this area, particularly high blood levels of serotonin, have been identified in a substantial number of autistic children. But too much vitamin B6 can be harmful, and some parents complain about adverse side effects. Moreover, the research cited in support of vitamin therapy is not widely viewed as convincing, although a recent review of research on this subject concluded that vitamin B6 plus magnesium appears to have at least a short-term beneficial effect in reducing autistic behavior in some individuals (Pfeiffer et al. 1995).

The Defeat Autism Now! (DAN!) conference held in early 1995 was convened by Bernard Rimland. About thirty medical researchers participated by invitation. A report on state-of-the-art alternative medical approaches to the treatment of autism, representing a consensus of the participants, was one outcome of the conference. Suggested interventions included intravenous immunoglobulin, antifungal medication, and gluten- and casein-free diets. (Gluten is a substance found in wheat and some other grains, and casein is a milk protein.) Each intervention was tied to the identification of a biological problem, with immune system dysfunctions and their effects highlighted.

A substantial number of parents reported marked decreases in their children's autistic behavior after the removal of milk products from their diets, and increases in such behavior with the reintroduction of milk. Mary Callahan, nurse and mother, was certain that her son's allergy to cow's milk was at the root of his autistic behavior or, minimally, exacerbated that behavior. She also believed that the elimination of milk products from his diet opened the door to his recovery. There is some evidence from research studies to support the idea that casein and gluten may contribute to the autistic behavior of some individuals.

The flyer from a local chapter of a disability agency announced a February 1996 presentation by a researcher, William Shaw, Ph.D. The caption read, "Could fungal or bacteriological infections be involved in your child's attention deficit disorder or autism?" The flyer went on to ask, "Could your ADD/autistic child benefit from dietary changes and antifungal medication?" As with all alternative treatments, not enough good research has been done to convince most medical researchers and other medical specialists concerned with autism that elevated levels of fungi or bacteria are involved in autistic behavior, or that the treatments being recommended will make a substantial difference in the learning or behavior of a significant number of individuals with autism. Yet many parents are placing their young children on "antifungal" diets (or are trying to), and some children are being given the antifungal medication nystatin.

There is increasing evidence of immune system abnormalities in autism. A substantial number of reports of research on this subject have appeared in medical journals since the 1980s, and most of these articles present data that appear to support the theory of a connection between immune system dysfunction and some cases of autism. The DAN! conference report states that the prevalence of immune system abnormalities has been found to be higher in individuals with autism than in the general population. Many parents are paying substantial sums of money for immunological evaluations and follow-up treatment. One recommended treatment commonly associated with such testing is intravenous immunoglobulin therapy (IVIG). While the value of this treatment is still questioned by many in the medical community, study of immune system abnormalities in autism has attained the status of mainstream medical research. The Seaver Center for Autism Research and Treatment, which was established in 1993 with a five-million-dollar foundation grant to Mt. Sinai Hospital in New York City, has identified immune system functioning as one of its areas of study. Mt. Sinai Hospital is a high-status medical center not particularly associated with alternative medicine.

Another alternative treatment championed by Bernard Rimland is auditory integration training (AIT), developed by the French otolaryngologist Guy Berard in the 1960s. (Another method of auditory integration training is in use, the Tomatis method, which was named after another French otolaryngologist whose work preceded Berard's.) Berard claims that he used AIT to treat almost 2,000 persons with learning/behavior disorders and 48 autistic individuals and that all of them benefited from this treatment to one degree or another. In a study of 445 children and adults with a primary or secondary diagnosis of autism, Rimland and Edelson (1994) found that auditory integration training reduced sound sensitivity and decreased problem behavior as reported by parents. But since no control or comparison group was used in this study, many researchers still remain skeptical about the benefits of this intervention strategy.

AIT was made popular in the United States by the publication of a book written by the mother of an autistic girl. "A miracle," is the way Annabel Stehli described her daughter's response to AIT, and the 1991 book in which this mother described what happened is called *The Sound of a Miracle*. Georgiana Stehli was diagnosed as autistic just before age three and entered an intensive educational treatment program at Bellevue Hospital a few months later. Annabel Stehli noted good progress in her daughter after several months of this treatment. She saw progress again when Georgie moved to a residential treatment center where the other girls, disturbed but not autistic, lured her out of her solitary world. Still, at age eleven Georgie was considered to be of borderline intelligence and too vulnerable and dangerous to live at home. Life in a residential setting was what professionals envisioned as Georgie's future. It wasn't a future her mother wanted any part of, so when she learned of a treatment for children with hyperaudition that held out the possibility of "recovery," Annabel Stehli pursued it. She noted signs of improvement almost immediately after the brief treatment period. For the first time Georgie wasn't afraid of certain sounds like the wind or ocean waves or even people's voices. "The rain didn't sound like a machine gun anymore," Georgie stated in a television interview. She wanted to go out and play, began to make new friends easily, and began to take pleasure in conversation. Although much remained to be done, Georgie now wanted to become normal, asked for instruction in achieving this goal, and soaked up the instruction her mother gave her. Her IQ, which had been seventy-five a year earlier, was now ninety-seven. Annabel Stehli felt that Georgie had been rescued.

What exactly is the treatment process that purportedly led to this dramatic improvement? And what was its effect on others with autism? The premise of AIT is that some of the characteristics of autism are a result of a sensory dysfunction and may involve hypersensitivity at certain sound frequencies, making some common sounds very painful to the autistic individual. (According to Bernard Rimland, about 49 percent of autistic children have symptoms of sound sensitivity.) In AIT a child or adult listens to modulated music through headphones for two half-hour periods a day over ten days, with certain sound frequencies filtered out. Why this should result in improved functioning is not clear. Berard believed that AIT enabled a person to adapt to intense sounds, but many other explanations have been proposed.

Annabel Stehli believes so strongly in AIT that she has devoted herself to spreading the word about this treatment through the Georgiana Organization, which was established for this purpose. There are many AIT success stories told by parents, stories of improvements in the comprehension of speech, in articulation, in the use of speech, and in focused attention; but most families don't experience a miracle or anything approaching it. Berard never claimed that faulty hearing was *the* cause of autism or that AIT is *the* treatment for it. Hearing is only part of the problem in autism, he wrote. But improved auditory functioning can go a long way toward helping the autistic child participate more fully in the major activities of living, some parents would add.

Data collected from parents on the outcomes of AIT include some reports of increased behavioral disturbances that disappear after a few days or weeks, along with many reports of decreased sound sensitivity and improved language and sociability. But one factor complicating the evaluation of AIT is that it is rarely the only alternative treatment parents use with their children. Often AIT accompanies two or three other alternative treatments such as megavitamin therapy, special diets, and sensory integration therapy, along with educational intervention.

Studies of AIT suffer from various limitations like the absence of control groups that leave positive claims for this treatment open to challenge. Thus, AIT is still considered a process in need of systematic study. Yet researchers are beginning to connect reports of sensory hypersensitivity by parents and by adults with autism to data on the functioning of the neurological system in autistic individuals. In commenting on this subject at a 1996 conference on autism, Martha Denckla, a neurologist from Johns Hopkins University School of Medicine who has long been involved in the study of neurologically based childhood disorders, voiced the view that alternative treatments like AIT and sensory integration therapy are closer to the cause of autism than are behavioral approaches. Moreover, a rigorously controlled research study, while finding that the electronically altered music used in AIT was no more effective than a structured listening program of unaltered music of wide frequency ranges and variety, concluded that both listening programs led to significant improvements in children with autism or Asperger's syndrome and signs of auditory distress (Bettison 1996).

Sensory integration therapy may be thought of as an intervention approach that parallels AIT but that focuses on other types of sensory input. It is one of the major treatment approaches or strategies used by occupational therapists—health professionals who treat children and adults with motor and sensory motor problems. Sensory integration therapy is widely used in programs for autistic children, many of whom are assessed as having sensory motor difficulties. Nonetheless, researchers like Gina Green, director of research at the New England Center for Autism (now the New England Center for Children), are skeptical about the value of sensory integration therapy, citing multiple weaknesses in the design of studies reporting positive results. "Well-controlled studies found that Sensory Integration Therapy was ineffective or no more effective than other treatments," she reports (1996, 24). Why then is this form of treatment used so widely? One reason is that it seems intuitively right.

No one who read Temple Grandin's first book (*Emergence: Labeled Au-*

tistic) or heard this adult with a Ph.D. speak of her childhood and adolescence will ever forget about the machine she developed to calm and
quiet herself. Her Squeeze Machine, modeled after a cattle chute, applies
firm pressure to the sides of the person's body, with the degree of pressure controlled by the person using it. Temple Grandin obtained a sense
of relief and relaxation as well as pleasurable tactile stimulation when
she was in this machine.

Kenneth was the five-year-old boy who was standing on his head
when I met him (see beginning of chapter 1). It was his favorite position,
his mother told me, one that he kept going back to as often as was allowed. And, she added, he seemed to be more responsive after one of
his head-standing periods. Other autistic children seem to crave movements like whirling or being swung around; and the use of mini-
trampolines is rewarding enough to serve as a reinforcer in some behavioral programs.

The tactile defensiveness of many young children with autism will
always remain clear in the minds of their parents: the infant who arches
his back and cries in response to his mother's attempts to hold him; the
aversion to being hugged or kissed or even touched. "Did you ever hear
of a kid who didn't like piggyback?" William Christopher had asked
plaintively, with his mind's eye on his own son. Even the refusal of some
autistic children to keeping their clothes on may be a defensive response
to sensitivity to certain textures, as explained by some adults with autism. Something is amiss here, sensory integration theory would indicate, some dysfunction in the proprioceptive, vestibular, and tactile systems.

The proprioceptive system receives sensory information from our
own bodies, specifically from the muscles and joints involved in movement. The vestibular system is responsive to gravity and to head movements, and it plays a role in awareness of body position, movement in
space, and balance. According to sensory integration theory, when the
information from the vestibular, proprioceptive, and tactile systems is
not integrated, the outcome will be poor body awareness, attention, and
motor planning, as well as other developmental problems. Sensory integration therapy addresses this dysfunction through sensory stimulation
and sensory motor challenges in activity contexts that are designed to

elicit adaptive behavior. Deep pressure, massage, vibration, and the use of play equipment like scooter boards, inclines, tunnels, swings, and sit-in toys that spin or rock are all commonly involved in sensory integration therapy.

Sensory integration therapy is not meant to be the only therapy that an autistic child receives. It is often integrated into an educational treatment program or is adjunctive to it; and parents of preschool children often arrange for this treatment along with speech services. Is this a waste of time, as the researcher Gina Green believes? Or are the parents who have found this a helpful facilitative approach correct? Clearly, more research on this subject is needed. Sensory integration therapy may not benefit many autistic children, but if I were a mother of an autistic child who appeared to have poor body awareness and coordination, who displayed tactile defensiveness, or was extremely fearful of activities that provided sensory motor challenges, I would certainly want my child to have sensory integration therapy. What I would try very hard to ensure is that this therapy did *not* cut into the intensity of my child's educational treatment.

There are undoubtedly many additional alternative treatments being used with autistic children. Some of these I have not referred to because their use has declined or has weak support; others because they have not (yet?) received a great deal of attention, use, or study. Some interventions that are beginning to attract more attention deal with visual functioning. Since many autistic children appear to have good visual skills, parents haven't often looked in this direction when they are searching for useful treatments; but some research data point to problems in this area, such as overfocused visual attention and difficulty in shifting attention. Moreover, both adults with autism and parents have reported that some problems in visual functioning are ameliorated by intervention techniques such as the use of special lenses.

"Breaking the Silence" was the title of an article in the August 1992 issue of *Teacher Magazine*. "Keyboard Helps Autistic Youths Find Their Voices, Advocates Say" was the name of another one in the June 11, 1992 issue of *Education Week*. "A History of Facilitated Communication: Science,

Pseudoscience, and Antiscience" appeared in the September 1995 issue of *American Psychologist*. "A request for information about facilitated communication," was the subject of a January 30, 1996 joint memorandum from an assistant secretary in the U.S. Department of Education and a commissioner in the Department of Health and Human Services. Facilitated communication (FC) had undoubtedly become the most controversial intervention approach used with autistic individuals in the 1990s, and probably one of the most reviled and maligned. It produced both hardened believers and hardened antagonists, with the weight of prestigious institutions increasingly behind those who cried "fraud." Gina Green referred to it as the single most harmful treatment introduced for autism.

In 1991 and 1992 facilitated communication was touted by the popular media as a miraculous way of opening up new worlds of possibility for people with autism. Article after article reported stories of children previously considered severely retarded who were typing meaningful and, in some cases, sophisticated ideas. The story below, which appeared in the *New York Times*, was typical.

> At the Donald R. Ray Middle School in Baldwinsville, N.Y., 14-year-old Lucy Harrison seems eager to spend her speech-therapy session talking to a reporter. Although from time to time she says "yes" aloud, she converses primarily by typing with her left index finger on a small black portable typewriter. Her speech therapist, Kate Walsh, sits beside her, with her right hand gently supporting Lucy's forearm halfway between the elbow and wrist, her thumb resting on top and her four fingers underneath the arm, as though ready to catch it. Lucy rapidly taps out sentences, ignoring typographical errors in her haste.
>
> As recently as 1989, Lucy was working at a first-grade level in a special-education classroom. This year, she was taking science, language arts and health in regular seventh-grade classes. Her most recent IQ tests place her in the high normal range, a leap of about 60 points, because she can now show her true abilities during testing. Without facilitation, Lucy types, "I would be helpless once again and it would be like a naked death." (Makarushka 1991, 70)

Yet by 1994 the picture had changed sharply, and what had been accepted as unrecognized ability was increasingly viewed as the communication of adult facilitators. Charges of "charlatanism" were hurled at the professionals promoting or implementing facilitated communication. But facilitated communication had not suddenly appeared without any foundation; in fact, this approach has deep roots in observations of the behavior of autistic children and in early treatment strategies.

Thirty years ago Dr. Mary Goodwin and her husband showed us that autistic children who don't communicate through speech may have unrecognized abilities. Mary and Campbell Goodwin were experienced pediatricians in the 1960s when they became interested in children with communication disorders. In their attempts to help such children they began using and testing the Edison Responsive Environment (E.R.E.), a cubicle containing a "talking typewriter" and programming device. The E.R.E. was made available for half-hour periods, one to five times a week, to each of sixty-five children diagnosed as autistic, as well as to children with physical disabilities and learning disabilities. Among the first children to be referred to the psychiatric clinic where the E.R.E. was located was a five-year-old boy with autistic behavior who had been excluded from kindergarten and was awaiting institutional placement. The Goodwins report the following observations:

> We invited Robbie's mother to bring him to the center for a trial of the E.R.E. He was led to the door of the booth with the words "Here is a typewriter for you." When Robbie went home 15 minutes later, he had left behind him a full page of random typing interspersed with many words, "liquid," "final," "touch," "ivory," "downy," "chlorox". . . .
> At later visits, he . . . wrote an original story paraphrased from "The Flintstones." (Goodwin and Goodwin 1969, 559–60)

Robbie was not the only child who demonstrated unexpected literacy on the typewriter. The Goodwins interpreted their findings to mean that the E.R.E. served to demonstrate abilities not tapped by conventional testing. The conclusion by the Goodwins that some autistic individuals have cognitive abilities that go unrecognized because they lack a means to express what they know is one of the central tenets of facilitated communication. This belief is not surprising if we consider that many autistic children don't communicate through speech or acquire speech much later than normally developing children and that some children diagnosed as autistic have nonverbal IQs in the normal range.

Facilitated communication differs from what occurred in the Goodwins' project in that it involves physical support from an adult who serves as a "facilitator."

> Facilitated communication is a means by which many people with major speech difficulties point at letters on an alphabet board or typing device to convey their thoughts. It involves a facilitator who provides physical support to help stabilize the arm, to isolate the index finger if necessary, to pull back the arm after each selection, to remind the individual to maintain focus, and to offer emotional support and encouragement; the facilitator progressively phases out the physical support. (Biklen 1992, 243)

This "facilitation" is at the core of the controversy of facilitated communication. Why should such physical support be necessary? (Would more children have benefited from the use of the Edison Responsive Environment in the Goodwins' project if such physical support had been provided?) Special education teachers often use physical guidance or prompting in teaching students with significant disabilities, but such prompting is reduced or faded out as quickly as possible because independent communication, using augmented or alternative means when necessary, is clearly the goal.

Professor Douglas Biklen of Syracuse University, the person who observed the use of facilitated communication in Australia and promoted it in the United States, proposed the idea that some autistic individuals have a problem with "praxis," that is, they have a neurologically based problem with expression that affects speaking and other ways of communicating their words and ideas. He points to a variety of observations and reports over the years, including those of the Goodwins, to support this contention. For example, in her 1974 book, *Effective Teaching Methods for Autistic Children*, Rosalind Oppenheim, a teacher of autistic children who was also the mother of an autistic child, made some observations about expressive difficulties in autistic children.

> The autistic child is deficient, not only in the ability to imitate, but also in his ability to *initiate* new motor patterns. . . . We maintain that autistic children have an output problem, and are literally unable to consciously

and volitionally activate their hands in certain instances when it is necessary. (Oppenheim 1974, 37–38)

Oppenheim described the special supports she devised in assisting
some of her students with various forms of expression. In response to
one twelve-year-old student who had "major difficulty with writing,"
Oppenheim reported that in order to write at all he needed "the touch of
the teacher's finger on his hand, very lightly—not guiding, but merely
touching—to structure the task for him" (64). Another student, seventeen years old, "has been introduced to the touch system of typing; but
he types very slowly, and insists on being touched while he is typing"
(72). What Oppenheim was doing in the 1960s sounds very much like
what facilitated communication is designed to do, and her rationale
sounds very much like the one offered by Biklen almost twenty years
later.

A mother of a young boy with autism provides another example, in
quite a different context, of what could be thought of as a need for facilitation. "Jason would either pedal or steer [the bike], . . . but he could
perform both these tasks simultaneously only if I were touching his
shoulder (facilitated bike riding??)" (Jasinski 1995, 19).

Sally Rogers, of the University of Colorado Health Sciences Center, is
known for her work on imitation in autistic children. Normally developing infants are very good imitators, she notes, an observation that has
been made by many clinicians and researchers. But the autistic child,
she states, has a specific deficit in the ability to imitate movements and
sometimes sounds. In fact, she had found this deficit in the imitation of
movements even in some intelligent adults with autism. Why should
this be? she asks. We don't really know, but one of the major explanations is that "there may be an underlying motor dysfunction, or dyspraxia, which interferes with the capacity to imitate another's movement" (1996b, 133).

Motor functioning in children with autism is commonly assessed by
the study of motor imitation and by gait analysis. Abnormalities in gait
are common in children with autism (Teitelbaum et al. 1996). Support
for the idea of movement difficulties in autism comes also from anatomical studies. Postmortem examinations have identified abnormalities in

the cerebellum, which is centrally involved in motor performance (Bauman and Kemper 1994).

Anne Donnellan and Martha Leary, in their 1995 book *Movement Differences and Diversity in Autism/Mental Retardation*, propose that movement is an integral part of virtually all aspects of expression, and that movement disturbances (e.g., the inability to start, stop, combine, and switch actions) are central to autism. Movement disturbances, they say, mask competence and create an impression of mental retardation. One example they give to support this view is an unexpected finding in a research study with adolescents who had limited verbal skills. Interviewers were told to wait expectantly for as long as it took the adolescents to respond. The researchers were surprised to discover that all the teenagers were able to offer good conversational responses if the interviewers were patient enough to wait for them to reply, something that took fourteen seconds on average instead of the normal period of under two seconds. These teenagers could participate in conversations but needed more time to formulate a response to what the other person said.

We have a long history of treating individuals with movement and communication disorders as mentally retarded. When institutions for the mentally retarded began being dismantled in the mid 1970s it was discovered that many of the people in these institutions had cerebral palsy or multiple disabilities that interfered with the production of speech; but they were not mentally retarded, even after years of neglect and deprivation. Today, speech/language therapists routinely work on augmentative and alternative communication with children who have neuromotor disorders that interfere with the acquisition of speech. Augmentative and alternative communication, which may involve the use of picture cards and boards, sign language, typewriters, computers, and electronic devices with programming features as well as voice or print output, is a widely accepted strategy. It draws on the concept of making accommodations to the needs of individuals who cannot communicate in typical ways.

Facilitated communication may be considered a form of augmentative and alternative communication designed to accommodate the needs of individuals who are autistic (or otherwise disabled) and have dyspraxia. The terms "praxis," "dyspraxia," and "apraxia" are an integral part of the professional vocabulary of the field of occupational therapy, with "dyspraxia" used to refer to developmental disorders of motor planning that cause the child to have difficulty in carrying out skilled, nonhabitual motor actions. If we accept the idea that autism reflects a neurological dysfunction or difference that may affect the production of speech and other forms of expression, it seems to make sense that some of these children may need special supports to facilitate writing and typing as well as speech. But some researchers strongly challenge the application of the concepts of dyspraxia or apraxia to autistic children and their use as an explanation for the amazing results reported for facilitated communication.

Facilitated communication has an inherent danger that is less likely to plague other types of augmentative and alternative communication, namely that the facilitator's continuing physical support may result in a product representing the facilitator's ideas rather than those of the child or adult being assisted. This hazard, and the situations it has led to, explain why facilitated communication came to be widely viewed as a misguided and ineffective method or even as a hoax.

When I first learned of the work of Rosemary Crossley at the DEAL Communication Centre in Melbourne, Australia, I was quite excited. The approach she developed in working with people who had cerebral palsy and was now also using with some autistic individuals seemed like a breakthrough. It appeared to confirm the combination of hope, fantasy, and wish of many parents and teachers that some autistic children know more than they can show. I even wrote to Professor Biklen and congratulated him on his role in bringing the facilitated communication strategy to the attention of professionals in the United States. But a few months after Douglas Biklen began offering training in facilitated communication, I attended a workshop in New York City given by a special education teacher who had been trained at Syracuse University and had been using FC with her students. I came away from that workshop very uneasy. The workshop leader was highly enthusiastic about FC. Too enthusiastic? I asked myself. Facilitated communication was the answer in the air, and almost everyone seemed to be jumping on the bandwagon. FC had revived the concept of autism as a shell or cage that prevented the person inside from showing his or her true capabilities. Parents and professionals very much wanted to believe that there might be a competent person inside waiting to express him- or herself.

Two factors played critical roles in turning opinion virulently against facilitated communication: multiple accusations of sexual abuse, usually against family members; and conclusions from studies using conventional research designs which found that facilitators were the source of the messages being produced in most instances. Sexual abuse is often difficult to confirm. The testimony of the abused individual may be the only evidence available. When awareness of the possibility of facilitator influence became widespread, public and professional opinion sided strongly with the accused families. Given the uncertainty of the situation, this outcome is easy to understand: some of the accusations were probably false and quite damaging to families. And yet the case of Darla (Brantlinger et al. 1994), a fifteen-year-old nonverbal autistic woman who was made pregnant by her fourteen-year-old brother in an apparently well functioning family, illustrates the fact that unlikely events do occur in the lives of individuals with autism. The high rate of abuse, both physical and sexual, of individuals with disabilities has been documented for almost a decade.

What even ardent promoters of FC do not dispute is that in some cases facilitators are determining the content of the typed communications. The issue that remains is whether facilitator influence on content is an aberration or whether it is endemic to FC and accounts for virtually all the unexpected findings of literacy in autistic individuals. If the communications being produced are largely authored by facilitators, then we have to reexamine the functions and methodology of FC itself.

The voice of the opponents of FC is well represented by a 1995 article in *The American Psychologist*, the major journal of the American Psychological Association. The authors of this article report that "the findings of controlled, as opposed to qualitative, studies have been consistently negative, indicating that . . . the content of the communication is being determined by the facilitator" (Jacobson et al., 754). Facilitators were unknowingly and unintentionally determining or influencing the messages being produced. Facilitated communication is "a pseudoscientific phenomenon," they concluded (759).

Proponents of FC have criticized "objective studies" in a variety of ways, some justified, others probably less so. One of the more justified criticisms is the assumption of almost all of these studies that if an individual can do something, for example, express his own ideas through typing, he will always be able to do it. Those who have worked with autistic individuals tell us that this is a highly questionable assumption. The records of many autistic students point to erratic and inconsistent performance, and Temple Grandin and other adults with autism have reported that during particular periods of childhood they could speak sometimes but not at other times. Proponents also point out that some individuals previously severely communication disabled can communicate independently after working with FC. Unfortunately, the number of autistic persons who have used FC but now type independently, while continuing to demonstrate the same level of literacy and sophisticated thinking, appears to be very small.

Where does that leave us? Is facilitated communication totally without value? Is it doing harm? The political fallout from the ascendance of these conclusions is that some service providers have withdrawn access to FC. Is this a good thing? One type of harm that FC may do is to keep children with autism from having intensive experiences with potentially more useful forms of augmentative and alternative communication. Another possible type of harm is that teachers and parents may stop trying to develop literacy skills because FC leads them to believe that the individuals they're trying to help already have those skills, even when they don't. Yet withdrawing access to FC altogether is a drastic step. It could cut off a channel of expression for those autistic individuals, however small their number, who do have complex ideas they can't otherwise express.

Moreover, the process of FC appears to engender desirable behavior—decreases in aggression and increases in on-task behavior—in some people with autism. Donnellan and Leary report that autistic individuals who are typically "uninterested in social interaction, easily distracted, in need of behavioral control techniques . . . are actually participating in a social interaction with no obvious external motivation except for the activity, the interaction itself" (1995, 94), and some of them are doing this for hours at a time. Something good appears to be happening in the FC process for some individuals with autism.

Rather than totally dismiss FC, we should try to figure out how to use it for what it can do for different individuals: serve as a mode of expression for some, as a learning mode for others. We could learn how to use it better, particularly in relation to the process of facilitation— searching for ways to deal more effectively with any dyspraxia that may be present so that dependence on a facilitator does not become chronic. We could figure out what brings about the desirable changes in behavior observable when some individuals engage in the process called facilitated communication and then try to extend these behavioral changes to other times, activities, and situations. While the concept of a cognitively competent, literate individual trapped inside a facade of autism is undoubtedly relevant to far fewer individuals than the initial reports on facilitated communication made it appear, we ought not be in the business of cutting off access to any approach that may be useful to some people with disabilities, even when that approach does not hold the whole answer we hoped for. Autism remains a puzzling condition. Given the great diversity of the autistic population, why can't we consider the idea that some autistic people may know much more than they can communicate, while others may know very little more than the fragments they show us?

This is also not the time to throw out the notion behind facilitated communication. Facilitated communication as this methodology is currently practiced may be in serious need of reexamination and repair, but it is a response to what increasingly appears to be a real and significant problem that some individuals with autism experience. Here is one recommendation of the working group on brain mechanisms of the National Institutes of Health's 1995 conference on the state of the science in autism:

> Reports of abnormalities in higher order motor abilities (praxis) and higher order cortical sensory abilities are now emerging. These findings may provide a basis for some of the unexplained aspects of the clinical

syndrome of autism such as the sensory distortions . . . and movement disorders. Apraxis could provide a neurologic explanation for the inability of very young autistic children to use sign language. Sensory and motor abnormalities may be quite disabling and intervention depends on a better understanding of the neurologic basis of these behavioral difficulties. There is a related need for research on movement and synchrony, building on some previous research in this area and on new findings in Parkinson's disease and autism. (Denckla 1996, 140)

As long as there are children—or adolescents or young adults—who are not developing in the typical way for reasons unknown to us, and as long as there is no known cure or highly effective treatment to make all of them function in typical ways, there will be alternative treatments and procedures designed to achieve this goal. Sometimes autistic individuals will be helped by these interventions, and sometimes they won't be. We can't stop parents from having a dream and trying to make it come true; nor should we try to do so.

part three Looking for Cures, Recovery, and Better Lives

9 Recovery?

One evening I was sitting in the rear of an almost empty bus when I noticed a young man walking toward the back of the bus and casually observed him. Something about him was familiar, I suddenly realized. When he sat on a seat adjacent to mine, I was sure. "Are you Victor W.?" I asked. "Who are you? How do you know me?" he replied.

Victor had been a student in my class seventeen years earlier. He was ten years old the last time I'd seen him. How did I recognize him? What first made him appear familiar was his walk, sometimes referred to as toe walking. It was less pronounced than when he was a child but still noticeable. The second memory trigger was his partial smile, not a communicative smile, not meant for anyone else. What made me sure it was Victor, the same Victor I described in chapter 6, was the mouth movements—tiny, rudimentary word formations that accompanied his thinking.

When Victor left my class and the treatment center in which it was located, he went to a small private school. We had all worked hard to help him make

*that transition. Now, after some initial discomfort at my mention of how I
knew him, Victor joyfully told me about his adult life. He was a doctoral student in an area of science. I remembered that his parents had wanted him to be
a doctor and that the head of the treatment team had referred to this wish as
evidence of the father's tenuous acceptance of Victor's condition. He did, in
fact, try to get into medical school, Victor told me, but wasn't accepted. He
was married now, Victor reported, and he told me about his wife's work. As
his stop approached, Victor gave me a warm good-bye and departed. We had
talked for almost twenty minutes.*

I was amazed and elated over this encounter. I remembered Victor as
he entered my class after five years of treatment. He had an excellent
memory and a large store of information, but his thinking was concrete
and rigid, and any unanticipated event could throw him into a frenzy.
For a year we worked on abstracting and generalizing, adapting and
coping, self-monitoring and self-control. I felt cautiously optimistic that
he would succeed in his regular education class, which had only eight
students in it because the school had just opened, but never did I anticipate that someday he would become a Ph.D. candidate. As soon as I
arrived home that evening I checked the telephone directory. His name
was there, and just seeing it there, the concreteness and certainty of it,
increased my elation, just as concreteness and certainty had made Victor
feel secure many years earlier.

A year or two later, I saw a notice in a university newsletter under
the heading "Alumni News." It was about Victor W., Ph.D., and gave
his workplace and title—along with the name of an article he wrote that
had just been published in a journal. A number of years have passed
since my chance meeting with Victor, but each year in that same newsletter I see Victor's name listed under alumni donors to the university
fund.

Had Victor recovered? Possibly. It depends on what is meant by recovery.

That word "recovery," the rallying cry of parents of young children with
autism who believe in Lovaas and Catherine Maurice, a word otherwise
unheard in relation to autism, is a word with an implied promise: nor-

malcy. Your child can be normal. How did this word enter the dictionary of autism when most highly regarded professionals view autism as a lifelong disorder (e.g., Lord and Rutter 1994, 578; Baron-Cohen 1995, 60)?

There have always been claims that children with autism have overcome that condition and have begun to function normally but, until Lovaas reported his treatment outcomes in 1987, these were isolated claims about a tiny percentage of autistic individuals. Let's examine various possible meanings of this claim of recovery. Does recovery mean that possible neurobiological factors underlying autism—differences in the structure or functioning of the brain, for example—have been eliminated? Or does it mean that while these neurobiological differences still exist, the impairments in behavior that reflected them have been reduced so significantly that the individual no longer meets the criteria for autism or any other developmental disability, although he or she continues to exhibit odd behavior and unusual adaptive strategies? Or does it mean that the individual's functioning is no longer distinguishable from what is considered typical or normal?

No one claims to have eliminated the neurobiological factors that may give rise to autism, although it is conceivable that intensive early learning experiences might cause alterations in the neurological system. Since we don't know what factors underlie autism, we can't assess changes in them. This takes us to the second and third possible definitions of recovery. Let's look at these definitions, applying them to Temple Grandin. Some people, impressed with her Ph.D., work success, writing, and presentations, might think of Temple as recovered, but she considers herself autistic. She has developed her own personal catalogue of strategies to deal with common situations that she found particularly difficult, so that for the most part she manages her life quite well. Yet she clearly differs from most people in the way she has to deal with such basic functions as learning, thinking, and remembering; she still has unusual difficulty in coping with certain types of social-affective interactions, such as those involved in casual dating or romantic relationships; and she has only recently begun to have what most people would consider real friendships.

After the publication of her 1995 book, Temple participated in book signings. One of them took place at a meeting of a local chapter of the Autism Society of America at which Temple was to make a presentation. When I entered the auditorium I saw Temple standing with her back to the wall near a table stacked with books. At the other side was a publisher's representative. Temple spoke neither to him nor to any of the people who came for her signature. When I brought her my copy I tried to begin a conversation, pointing out that I had purchased her book earlier and had read it thoroughly, as she could see from the slips sticking out of it at various places. There was no response from Temple. She silently signed her name, nothing more. Later, during her animated and impressive presentation, she mentioned that she never wrote anything but her name in her book because she didn't know what else to write.

In his book *An Anthropologist on Mars* Oliver Sacks has this to say about the question of recovery in relation to Temple Grandin: "'Normality' had been revealed more and more, as we spoke, as a sort of front, or facade, for her, albeit a brave and often brilliant front, behind which she remained, in some ways, as far 'outside,' as unconnected, as ever" (1995, 275).

Catherine Maurice's children no longer meet the criteria for autism, but have their impairments in communication and social functioning been eliminated, or are these children achieving generally normal outcomes by different routes? Have all their impairments truly gone away, or will differences in coping mechanisms show up later in their development? Before the question of recovery can be examined productively, an operational definition has to be specified.

The mother of the university graduate mentioned in chapter 2 told the audience waiting to hear her son's presentation, "My son and I have both rediscovered his autism. He was diagnosed as autistic as a child, and then the label was removed, and we thought he used to be autistic; but now we know he is autistic." The term "recovered" doesn't fit her son well. There are a good number of adults with autism who look normal in many ways, but who still feel different and still have difficulty dealing with some basic aspects of everyday life.

Since the recent use of the term recovery stems primarily from the claims of Lovaas, let's look at how he defines this term. In his 1987 article "Behavioral Treatment and Normal Educational and Intellectual Functioning in Young Autistic Children"—which caught the attention of the academic world—Lovaas reported that nine out of nineteen children who participated in his intensive behavioral treatment program had achieved normal functioning by age seven (although one of these nine children was removed from this category when a later follow-up study found that he had been placed in a special education class). The term "recovered" is used a couple of times in that article to refer to these nine children. By normal functioning Lovaas meant having an IQ in the average range (or better), being maintained in regular classes, and being promoted from grade to grade. Lovaas did, however, acknowledge that some children can meet this definition of normal functioning and still have residual deficits that may become obvious only as a child gets older. Like the university graduate who lost his autism label in childhood only to reclaim it later. But the recovery claims that Lovaas makes go beyond the operational definition used in 1987. In a film showing five boys who had been part of his Young Autism Project, three of them identified here as having recovered, Lovaas essentially challenges the viewer to distinguish two of these adolescents from the friends with whom they are shown. Indeed, on the basis of the brief film footage provided, I could not make this discrimination.

The follow-up study reported in 1993 added other measures to assess whether the nine children considered to have normal functioning had residual deficits. It used the Vineland Adaptive Behavior Scales, the Personality Inventory for Children, and a clinical interview. While Lovaas and his associates (John McEachin and Tristram Smith) concluded that eight of the children did not have residual deficits, this conclusion was questioned by reviewers like Peter Mundy of the University of Miami (1993). Mundy pointed out, for example, that there were insufficient reliability and validity data for the clinical rating scale and that parent report measures such as the Vineland and the Personality Inventory for Children, while good at identifying external forms of disturbance, are not as good at identifying the unusual thought processes and internalized forms of disturbance likely to be characteristic of high-functioning individuals with autism. Thus, Mundy counseled caution in accepting the follow-up data as sufficient proof of completely normal functioning or recovery. Nonetheless, these adolescents appeared to have achieved essentially normal functioning.

What is the future for autistic individuals? How do most autistic children turn out or fare as adults? This is the broader context into which questions about recovery should be placed. The answer to the question of outcomes can best be obtained from follow-up studies of autistic children who have reached adolescence or adulthood. An analysis of eight early follow-up studies found a common pattern: from 5–17 percent of autistic children had good outcomes, while 61–74 percent had poor or very poor outcomes, and the remainder had fair outcomes (Lotter 1978). The definition of "good outcome" used in this analysis was normal or near-normal social life along with satisfactory functioning at school or work. This definition is not equivalent to recovery, but it would include instances of recovery.

Perhaps the most interesting of the early follow-up studies are those done by Leo Kanner (1973). Twenty-eight years after the appearance of his ground-breaking 1943 article on autism, a follow-up study was done of the children described in that publication. Eight of the eleven children from the original study participated in the follow-up. Kanner found that two of them had good outcomes, and one of these two had achieved very close to normal functioning. He was a college graduate who did well at his job as a bank teller. He also belonged to a variety of organizations, including a local Kiwanis club, where he had served a term as president. Even so his mother, while very proud of his accomplishments, described him as not completely normal; he did not express his inner feelings, rarely participated in social conversation, showed no interest in the opposite sex, and displayed little initiative (Kanner 1973).

Another study reexamined forty-two children diagnosed as autistic by Leo Kanner. Only one of these individuals could be considered to have achieved normal functioning. He was married and a father, had served as a meteorologist in the navy for two years, and had achieved some success in composing music.

A third follow-up report on autistic children seen at Johns Hopkins Hospital, where Kanner was based, involved ninety-six children. This study identified nine additional individuals with good outcomes, with the criteria for good outcome being employability, absence of obvious behavior problems, and satisfactory social relationships. Of these nine, four had college degrees, two were attending college, and three were employed full time. None of the nine had married, but five of them lived independently and several were dating.

The results of a large follow-up study done at the University of Indiana Medical School were generally consistent with Kanner's findings. Ten percent of the autistic children had either good or very good outcomes, and two of them were considered normal in all respects at follow-up. Of these two, Candace, whose performance IQ at age three was 108, was considered normal by age seven. Alfred, who wasn't considered normal until age twelve, had a performance IQ of 62 at age three, at which time he was also highly withdrawn and nonverbal; but Alfred was the highest functioning individual in the follow-up sample. He was an A student and was active in student affairs (DeMyer et al. 1973).

None of the studies just described reported anything like the percentage of children apparently achieving normal functioning in the Lovaas program, but treatment was not a major variable in any of these studies, and intensive treatment of any kind was rarely available. However, in the late 1960s Kanner conducted a follow-up study of children who had been involved in an intensive treatment program at the Linwood Children's Center in Maryland. Linwood was a center founded by a teacher specifically for children considered psychotic, a good many of whom met Kanner's definition of autism. The center espoused an approach that stressed acceptance of the child and his behavior, and expansion of that behavior into more varied and functional activities. The treatment framework was developmental/psychodynamic. Kanner concluded that at least six of the fifteen autistic children he studied had achieved either full recovery or close to normal functioning. They did well in mainstream educational programs, had friends, and engaged in a variety of age-appropriate activities such as sports. While the treatment provided at this center was quite different from the behavioral approach used by Lovaas, the center's rate of normal or close to normal outcomes is considerably higher than the rate reported in other studies, and not much less than the recovery rate reported by Lovaas. This finding underscores the value of intensive educational treatment and supports the idea that interventions that differ significantly from the behavioral approach of Lovaas and his followers can result in good outcomes for a substantial number of children with autism.

A more recent study conducted in Toronto (Szatmari et al. 1989) focused on sixteen adults who had been treated at a center for autistic children under the age of six, and who had IQs above 65 at the time they were in treatment at that center. A major study finding was that the outcomes for this group were considerably better than outcomes reported in other studies that included children with lower IQs. Four of the adults would have been considered normal by most people unfamiliar with their childhood functioning. These four adults had IQs above 100 and had earned university degrees. They lived in their own apartments and needed no supervision. One of them, a student, was married; the other three held full-time jobs and also dated regularly. Thus, 25 percent of these autistic adults could be considered to have achieved essentially normal functioning. While the twelve other adults continued to have substantial problems in functioning, several had higher education degrees and three held jobs in the community. This study did not focus on the effects of treatment, but it may well be that the psychotherapeutic treatment all of these individuals received during early childhood also contributed to their better outcomes.

A study of seventy-six Canadian "third-generation" autistic children—individuals born between 1974 and 1984—found no significant change in IQ in this group over a period of about four years (Eaves and Ho 1996). The mean age of the children at the first testing was 7.1 and at the second testing was 11.6; the mean verbal IQ at both times was 58, while the mean performance IQ was 63 at the first assessment and 62 at later testing. Furthermore, all children continued to meet the criteria for autistic spectrum disorder, and only 7 percent of the children developed friendships. In light of the fact that all these children had been diagnosed before age five, had attended preschool, and were receiving special education support, the results of this study were disappointing.

However, only about 14 percent of the children were nonverbal. This finding would be more encouraging if the definition of verbal used in the study (having more than five words) were not so generous as to allow the inclusion of children who might have very limited communication skills. Functional speech has been the focus of many past studies that found this goal to be achieved by only half of autistic individuals. A somewhat hopeful finding was that the percentage of children with IQs in the range identified as mental retardation was lower than the estimate of 75 percent generally given in the past, the percentage found in this study being 53 percent if performance IQ was used and 62 percent if verbal IQ was used. Thus, while some general improvement of outlook was noted, the change was not dramatic.

A recent analysis of outcome studies concluded that whereas the vast majority of autistic children remain severely socially restricted in adulthood, a very small number of such children appear to "grow out of autism" and become cured or have extremely good outcomes. As older adolescents and adults they are indistinguishable or almost indistinguishable from nondisabled people (Gillberg 1991). This conclusion breeds both hope and fear in parents and other caring adults; hope that a particular child will be one of those who becomes an indistinguishable former autistic; and fear that the child may be one of the much larger proportion of autistic children who will remain severely socially restricted in later life.

What an analysis of follow-up studies does not give us is a blueprint for increasing the number of children who become indistinguishable from nondisabled people or almost so. During the past few years, earlier identification of autistic children and changes in federal education law have combined to make treatment of two- to four-year-old children with autism much more common. This change can be expected to lead to an increase in the percentage of autistic children who achieve good outcomes.

Anecdotal reports and case studies of recovery from autism have appeared in the literature from time to time over many years. They tell us a different part of the story of recovery. Perhaps the best publicized case of recovery is that of Raun Kaufman, whose father, Barry, has told this story many times in different forms. The story became well known through a book, *Son Rise*, that appeared in 1976, and a 1979 television movie based on this book. A revised version of the original book plus an update and additional case studies was published in 1994 under the title *Son Rise: The Miracle Continues.*

Even before their son's diagnosis, the Kaufmans thought "autism" and began a search for answers. They found none that satisfied them— not from Ivar Lovaas or Bernard Rimland or Bruno Bettelheim—and day-by-day they saw their infant son slipping away from them. Their answer? They would create their own path, their own way of accepting and reaching their gentle but distant child. They observed him intensively, looking for clues to ways of connecting and communicating with him. They joined him in his spinning and rocking rituals, trying to break into his world. His environment was simplified, and all his waking hours were spent with a parent or other caregiver, with about six hours a day spent in structured or semi-structured activities. Raun was seventeen months old when the program to help him began. A formal evaluation when he was twenty months old showed an autistic child whose language and social development was still like that of an infant of about eight months. The next evaluation, at twenty-four months, showed age-appropriate developmental levels in all areas.

Shortly after his first book appeared, I invited Barry Kaufman to address the course I had just introduced into the master's degree program in special education at Hunter College, "Working with Parents of Young Handicapped Children." He came. His son was five at that time and was in nursery school. In some ways Raun was functioning above his age level, Barry Kaufman told my students, but some unusual behavior was still present. He was very touch-oriented, for example, and if he saw a baby in a carriage he might go up to it and stroke its face, an action not usually viewed in a favorable light by the infant's mother. Barry Kaufman had no doubt, however, that his son would do fine in school and elsewhere.

About twelve years later I received some promotional material for the Option Institute that Barry Kaufman and his wife, Samahria (Suzi in his first book), had established in Sheffield, Massachusetts to teach their philosophy and approach to other families, professionals, and adults in general. In a brochure that was part of the packet, Raun was described as a ninth grader in a public school who had been a straight-A student for several years, who had an IQ of 150, who was highly gregarious, and who had no residual signs of autism.

In 1994 two additional pieces of information about Raun appeared in print. An article in *The New York Teacher*, the newsletter of the state teachers' union, described Raun as a senior at an ivy league college majoring in biomedical ethics; and Raun himself, in the foreword to his father's "new" book, informed us that he was on his college's debating team, loved Stephen King novels, wrote science fiction stories, had a girlfriend, drove a car, was studying ballroom dancing, and was a member of a fraternity. Recovered? It certainly seems so.

Several years ago I received a package at my college office. It came from the father of a five-and-one-half-year-old girl and held the manuscript of a book about his daughter's "successful struggle against autism." I called this father and talked to him about his daughter and the intervention process that he and his wife used. They had learned the approach at the Option Institute.

For four years I heard nothing about the book or the child, so I called again. The manuscript had not been published, the father reported; he decided that he didn't want his daughter to be known as the girl who had been autistic. She was now functioning like other children in all ways, he told me, except that she was two years behind in her development because of the time she had lost to autism. At age six she had entered a pre-kindergarten class instead of the first grade. Since then she had been progressing at the usual rate and was doing well in school. She had friends, was very well liked, and participated in neighborhood activities. How had this been achieved? I asked this father. By twelve hours of work, day in and day out, for four years, with the help of many volunteers, he replied. The treatment program had taken some time to begin working, but after two years his daughter was almost out of her autism; in four years there were no traces of autism left, he stated.

Yes, the Option Institute did charge a lot of money for the Son-Rise program, the father agreed, but it was worth it. Before they had gone to the Option Institute he had spent a couple of thousand dollars on specialists and had received no help. They had been at their wit's end, what with their daughter's tantrums, attacks on them, and the injuries she inflicted on herself. The Son-Rise program was certainly worth the money, this father told me, because it helped them rescue their child from autism and saved their family.

It's hard to describe exactly what the Son-Rise program is. Part of the reason for this difficulty is that Barry Kaufman doesn't think about intervention in the same way that most professionals in the field of autism do, and he doesn't use the same categories and labels to describe it. Another reason is that the only written descriptions of what occurs in this treatment approach come in the context of Raun Kaufman's story or a handful of vignettes about other children.

Still, certain aspects of what the Son-Rise model encompasses appear clear. The overall philosophy is that attitude matters a lot, and the attitude that helps is one of love and acceptance of the child, however he functions in both the present and the future. This attitude gets translated into an initial methodology very much in tune with the thinking of Stanley Greenspan, Geraldine Dawson, Barry Prizant, and other developmentally based theorists and therapists (mentioned in chapters 3 and 6). By mirroring their son's behavior and following his lead, the Kaufmans tried to entice him into noticing and interacting with them. The Son-Rise approach has other elements that fit current thinking, like its one-to-one in-home model involving many hours a week of interaction, and the use of multiple individuals (usually volunteers) to assist the family in implementing this intensive program.

The Son-Rise model has generated tremendous controversy largely because it breaks all the rules: it wasn't developed by professionals, isn't directed by someone with professional credentials in autism, describes its methods only in very broad terms, and doesn't collect or report outcome data in ways that are considered acceptable by the professional community. This last factor makes it difficult to judge how effective this approach is. It apparently led to an excellent outcome for Raun Kaufman and a few other children, but what about the many others whose families used it? According to Barry Kaufman, the Son-Rise approach has "facilitated deep-seated and lasting change in hundreds of children and their families" (1994, 245). Unfortunately, he does not define "deep-seated change" in terms of specific outcomes; therefore, we have no idea of how many of these hundreds of children achieved anything approaching normal functioning or even moderately good outcomes. "Deep-seated and lasting change in children and families" can mean that parents have come to accept their child's autism and its implications instead of being in a constant state of turmoil and conflict about it, as one mother who used this approach reported to me. A handful of case studies is the only outcome data reported. Kaufman is asking parents to take his word, to have faith in an approach that is skimpily described and has weakly documented outcomes, while paying a great deal of money in the process.

The previous chapter introduced Annabel Stehli and her daughter, Georgiana, champions of auditory integration training, to which the elder Stehli attributed Georgie's emergence from an autistic existence. Whatever the role that AIT played in Georgie's development, she has achieved what appears to be close to normal functioning. Her Bachelor of Fine Arts degree came magna cum laude, and she is married. Not long ago when Georgiana made a presentation at a conference, I searched for residual signs of autism. The presentation handout identified her as co-coordinator and illustrator on a curriculum project for autistic adolescents and adults. It also described her as an international speaker on her own autistic experiences, a consultant to a center for the study of autism, an illustrator and artist.

Georgiana Stehli Thomas is an attractive young woman who appeared poised during her presentation. I could identify only one act that might reflect a residue of Georgie's autism. When she was handed the microphone, Georgie announced that she felt ready to eat an ice-cream cone because that was what the mike reminded her of. While I could immediately empathize with this association, it was an unusual way to open a presentation; not bizarre, even charming in a way, but certainly not typical.

When questions were taken from the audience, Georgiana was asked: "What autistic characteristics do you still have?" She was still supersensitive to smells and hyposensitive to cold and heat, she replied. She swims in the frigid waters of Oregon for sixty to ninety minutes at a time; cold doesn't bother her at all. During the question and answer period that followed the presentation, one of the audience members called on was an autistic man, and he spoke at great length about his personal experiences. It was Georgie who responded to this situation, and she did so with gentleness and respect while getting the session moving again.

Now let's return to Ivar Lovaas's statements that have fueled a major controversy in the professional literature since the late 1980s. At dispute is his claim that the children who achieved the best outcomes have achieved normal functioning. Are these individuals recovered, or are they autistics with near-normal functioning? The average age of the individuals in the last follow-up study was thirteen. It may be that a more definitive answer to this question must await another study when most of these individuals have reached adulthood, and when a more comprehensive assessment of social functioning and flexibility in thinking is conducted.

Autistic individuals with near-normal functioning can and do graduate from college, have better than average IQs, and participate in some activities in the community; but they often have no close friends, don't date, have difficulty obtaining and holding jobs commensurate with their education and ability, and feel different from "typicals" in significant ways.

Drew Johnson is one of the successes of Ivar Lovaas's Young Autism Project. During his second year of college Drew wrote the afterword in his mother's book about his recovery. At one point Drew states:

> I do have trouble expressing my feelings to others. The main reason I believe is that I have a linear thought process. I don't know why I think like this because my mom, brother, and sister are very emotional. I do express my emotions in extreme cases. For example, when a family member dies or when one of my friends gets screwed. There is a good

side, however. The fact that I am not very emotional helps me in every decision I have to make. (Johnson and Crowder 1994, 182)

Personality difference or residue of autism or residue shading into personality?

An accumulation of evidence collected over more than thirty years from multiple sources shows that some individuals with autism do go on to enjoy an essentially normal life or something very close to it. Such individuals have had varying life experiences that are not associated with only one particular type of treatment. It is also clear that other autistic individuals have achieved lives that appear normal on casual viewing but not on closer scrutiny. The mother of a young adult with two master's degrees and a job as the manager of a developmental disabilities resource center wrote, in the introduction to a newsletter article by her son: "Jean-Paul is not 'cured.' He . . . still has problems related to his autism" (Bovee 1995, 6). The current motto of the Georgiana Organization is Progress—progress, not perfection.

Some parents and many professionals decry references to recovery or any other term that might be taken to imply that autism can be cured. They feel that such references are misleading and cruel, that they fuel hopes that will not be realized. Yes, it is true that there is no cure for autism, and many families will be disappointed when the treatments that reportedly produced individuals like Raun Kaufman or the Maurice children don't result in similar outcomes for their son or daughter. We need to be very careful about making any claims that will mislead parents, but we also need to take care not to wipe out their hopes. We need stories of triumph to show that all efforts are not futile, and we need other stories to show that even when recovery is not possible, individuals with autism are leading better lives—lives that have more satisfactions—than was ever possible in the past.

A parent asked, What if my son remains autistic? What will we do? The best you can—with your love, your skills, and all the resources you can marshal—to help him achieve as independent and joyful a life as is possible for him.

10 Moving Toward Better Answers

More than thirty years have passed since I was a teacher of Nellie, Sean, and other children with autism. If these children had been born after 1990 instead of before 1960, could I or others have helped them more? Could they have come more easily to understand the world around them and learned better ways to communicate their needs, desires, and ideas to others? Could Nellie's self-abuse have been avoided? Could Sean have reached a point where head banging was something in his past? Could they have gone to schools and been in classes with other children from their neighborhoods? It's impossible to answer these questions with any certainty, but Nellie and Sean would have a much better chance of reaching these markers of typicality today.

Why is this true? What has changed? Recognition of autism has changed. It's no longer a condition that's ignored or brushed aside until a child reaches age four or five. Autistic children are increasingly being diagnosed before age three, sometimes even before or around their second birthday. Society's attitude toward individuals with severe disabilities, including autism, has changed. We no longer believe that people who are very different in some ways need to be shut off from the world of "typicals." Autistic children are not sent to institutions, as Sean was, although a very small number reside in treatment centers for varying periods of time. The educational service picture has changed. It's no longer necessary to fight for education for an autistic child, or wait until an autistic child is five or six or even seven before he or she can go to school. Early intervention services are now available for infants and toddlers, and increasing numbers of two-year-olds with various types of pervasive developmental disorders, including autism, receive these services. Today children who go to special schools usually do so because their parents believe that they will receive more help there, not because no other options are available. And no teacher today is expected to be the sole adult in a classroom with five to eight autistic students, as I was in the early 1960s. How much more I could do for Nellie, I used to think, if only there were another adult in the classroom so that I could work alone with Nellie for chunks of time during the school day.

All of the above is true, but it's no guarantee that Nellie and Sean would do well, only that they would have a much better chance for a good life. We still don't know enough to help all the Nellies and Seans, and only a lucky few get the best of what we do know today about treating children with autism. Let's look at what we can do, need to do, if the Nellies and Seans of today are to have a better chance at a fuller life.

There are three major avenues for improving the lives of individuals with autism or eliminating autism from their lives altogether. The first is identification of the neurobiologic substrate(s) of autism and development of treatments to prevent or correct the deviation that leads to the behavioral syndrome called autism; in other words, to find a cure for autism. Until this is possible, we must pursue other avenues. Advances in the effectiveness of pharmacological treatment, education, and other behavioral interventions form the second major path toward improved lives for children and adults with autism. The third route involves

changes in policy and practice that will bring education and other publicly funded intervention services closer to the state of the art, so as to
provide greater equity in the matter of treatment.

What we are searching for ultimately are answers at the biological
level. Without understanding the causes and pathogenesis of autism,
the paths it takes from original difference or damage, we grope about in
semi-darkness. Still, this is an exciting time in biomedical research. Almost weekly, newspapers and magazines carry stories about breakthroughs in our understanding of how human biological systems operate, and what kinds of breakdowns in these systems lead to various
types of medical conditions and disorders in behavior.

The Human Genome Project, begun in 1990 under the direction of the
National Institutes of Health, is a comprehensive endeavor to "find the
location of 100,000 or so human genes" that make each of us unique
(Department of Health and Human Services 1995). The project will develop tools to help scientists find genes quickly, and therefore be better
able to identify the genes involved in diseases. It could lead to the identification of individuals genetically predisposed to certain conditions, to
the development of highly targeted drugs that would act on those genes,
and, eventually, to the replacement of such genes. Given the finding that
heredity appears to have a significant role in autism, the Human Genome Project is highly relevant to the search for causes and cures for
autism. No cures for autism loom on the immediate horizon, but this
goal is no longer only a dream for a very distant future.

In the meantime, studies of the neuropathology of autism are producing valuable clues to differences in brain structure and function in autistic as compared with nonautistic people. No longer are researchers looking for one brain structure or region that is grossly abnormal. Instead,
what is envisioned are multiple areas with subtle differences. Dr. Margaret Bauman, of the department of neurology, Massachusetts General
Hospital, has been studying the anatomy of the brain in autism for more
than a decade, using autopsy material from children and young adults
who died as a result of injury or illness. She has identified several differences in brain structure between individuals with autism and matched
controls. The limbic system of the brain is believed to play a major role

in emotion. The amygdala, part of the limbic system sometimes referred to as the brain's "emotional computer," appears to mediate several responses—motivation, attention, and representation—involved in social orienting, joint attention, and recognition of the affective significance of stimuli. Bauman found that neurons in the amygdala and other parts of the limbic system of individuals with autism are smaller and more densely packed than those in people without autism, perhaps because the early pruning of neurons that normally takes place has not occurred, leading to developmental curtailment. Such limbic system abnormalities might be involved in producing some of the core characteristics of autism.

Bauman has also identified abnormalities in the cerebellum, which is considered the coordinating center for movement and is thought to ensure optimal performance of voluntary motor acts. The cerebellum may also have a role in the modulation of sensory input, attention, emotion, and some aspects of language. Thus, abnormalities in the cerebellum may contribute to difficulties in learning, social interaction, and communication. Bauman has begun to study neuroanatomic material from individuals with Asperger's syndrome, and her preliminary findings are that the degree of abnormality in the limbic and cerebellar systems is more limited in individuals with this syndrome than in autism (Bauman 1996).

Findings from studies using magnetic resonance imaging (MRI) provide some support for the anatomical differences in the cerebellum identified by Margaret Bauman. Eric Courchesne, who pioneered the use of magnetic resonance imaging, has argued that the cerebellum ensures optimal performance of several neural systems, for example, the sensory and attentional systems, to which it is functionally connected. Thus, cerebellar abnormality could place the young autistic child on a developmental pathway that Courchesne and his associates refer to as "misorganizing" (1994). Such a pathway would be consistent with the reports of autistic adults about their fragmented and confusing experiences in childhood.

With autism now widely viewed as a disorder of neuronal organization, neuroimaging is increasingly being used to study individuals with this condition, and imaging research is beginning to produce important information about neural structures and mechanisms. Imaging studies have generally supported neuropsychological findings on autism. The frontal lobes of the brain have been identified as critical to planning, impulse control, organized problem solving, and flexibility in thinking and acting, areas in which many autistic individuals have difficulty. (These processes are often referred to as "executive functions.") Children with autism and either normal or near normal IQs perform significantly more poorly than do nonautistic children of the same mental age on neuropsychological tests designed to assess planning and flexibility in problem solving. Moreover, frontal lobe damage in childhood is known to impair the ability to understand the viewpoints of others and demonstrate appropriate empathy, characteristics often found in autistic persons. Some imaging studies using positron emission tomography (PET) have identified abnormal metabolism in the frontal lobes of individuals with autism, as well as in functionally related areas of the brain; and some EEG data appear to show that children with autism have less activity in the left frontal lobe, particularly in areas most closely linked to the limbic system, than do nonautistic children.

Very few studies have used PET to study children because this technology involves exposure to radiation. Functional magnetic resonance imaging (fMRI), a noninvasive method that emerged in the 1990s, will allow for expanded study of brain functioning in children. Neural activity is accompanied by changes in blood flow, blood volume, and blood oxygenation within the brain that show up on fMRIs. Thus, fMRIs can provide information about the localization of neural activity during various types of tasks or activities.

Neurochemicals are involved in multiple aspects of neural development, and abnormal brain chemistry has been identified in several conditions thought of as mental disorders. A number of studies have found abnormalities of the neurotransmitter serotonin in children and adults with autism. Since such abnormalities may be genetically based, the study of differences between autistic and nonautistic children in this and other neurochemicals may shed light on the pathophysiology of autism and lead to new and more effective treatments.

At present, no drug has been approved by the U.S. Food and Drug Administration specifically to treat autism. The drugs that are used with some autistic individuals act on selected behaviors found in both autism and comorbid conditions, for example, the rituals central to obsessive-compulsive disorders. Drugs are also used to reduce the anxiety, depression, or aggression that have been observed in some adolescents and young adults with autism. Some autistic children with epileptiform abnormalities on EEGs are being treated with anticonvulsants like valproic acid. While remission of core symptoms of autism has been reported for some children (e.g., by Plioplys 1994), not enough research has been done to determine whether this treatment will be effective with significant numbers of autistic children. Pharmacological treatment of autism has a long way to go.

Fortunately, support for research into the biomedical factors in autism has increased dramatically since 1995. Parents have played a major role in making this happen. The Autism Society of America, a parent-driven organization, wanted the National Institutes of Health to assume a more active role in research on autism. In order to achieve this objective, ASA devoted intensive advocacy efforts to gaining congressional support. Those efforts paid off. In April 1995 NIH held a working conference on the state of the science in autism research, a conference that served as a launching pad for more vigorous and coordinated efforts into research on autism.

Parents have been active in other research-support endeavors as well. The National Alliance for Autism Research (NAAR), based in Princeton, New Jersey, was formed in 1994 by a group of parents of autistic children. These parents were dismayed by the absence of a national organization on autism to compare with the Cystic Fibrosis Foundation, which had raised almost eighteen million dollars for research in 1994. They were also distressed by the fact that research on some conditions less prevalent or about as prevalent as autism received much more funding from NIH than did autism research. The goal of NAAR is to advance biomedical research into the causes, prevention, treatment, and cure of autistic spectrum disorders. In a short period of time NAAR designed several strategies for advancing autism research, established an impressive scientific advisory board to select projects for funding, and began fund-raising efforts. One of NAAR's strategies is to provide funding for pilot projects and postdoctoral research that would enable newer autism researchers and new types of research to compete more successfully for major NIH grants.

CAN, which stands for Cure Autism Now, is another group devoted to the support of biomedical research; its particular focus is research that appears to be closely linked to treatment. Founded in 1995 by two mothers of autistic children, one of them a pediatrician, this Los Angeles group seeks to accelerate progress by supporting "cutting-edge" research and by facilitating collaboration among researchers.

Now let's turn to the educational treatments we already have in place today, which were described in earlier chapters. Sally Rogers, in a summary of her presentation at the 1995 NIH research conference, pointed out that at least six comprehensive educational treatment programs with distinct curricula and strategies have published data in respected professional journals on positive treatment outcomes. What all these intervention programs had in common was a focus on very young children (ages two to four at the beginning of treatment) and on intensity of treatment in terms of hours per week, very low child-to-adult ratios, and continuation of treatment for a minimum of one to two years. Rogers concluded that if it were possible to achieve on a large scale the same positive treatment outcomes as these model programs have achieved, then "the typical education and treatment programs for young children with autism available in most communities need to be drastically redesigned and funded" (1996a, 246).

It is time to reexamine how we use public systems and funds to serve young autistic children. We need to begin directing public resources to those service models that give young children the best possible chance of overcoming the devastating effects of autism. Programs that don't offer them such a chance are not appropriate. While we can't realize all our dreams for helping autistic children, we can do much more than we are doing today. We can, for example, work on the following strategies:

Use state-of-the-art techniques to identify toddlers who appear to have autism or other pervasive developmental disorders. While some toddlers identified before the age of two may not look autistic at age three, research data show that all toddlers so identified show some kind of developmental delay or disability at age three (e.g., Baron-Cohen et al. 1996; Lord 1995). The infant/toddler section of IDEA, the federal education law focused on children with disabilities, calls for action aimed at early identification, but more strenuous efforts are needed. Furthermore, such efforts should be targeted particularly to low-income families and other families with inexperienced, isolated, and/or overburdened parents. These are the families in which autistic children are least likely to be identified early.

Provide intensive services to toddlers and preschoolers. The cost of intensive (one-to-one) services for every two-, three-, and four-year-old diagnosed as having autism or another pervasive developmental disorder would undoubtedly be extremely high. But the current, often feeble, attempts at intervention for this population are unlikely to reduce the even greater cost of maintaining a very large proportion of autistic individuals as seriously disabled throughout their lifetimes. It is cost-effective to help as many young autistic children as possible become part of the mainstream of society early in their lives, and we need intensive efforts to accomplish this.

Not every child diagnosed as having a pervasive developmental disorder needs thirty or forty hours a week of formal educational treatment services for an extended period of time; and some children who begin receiving intensive services at age two or three will, a year or two later, be able to learn effectively in small groups and benefit from supported participation in inclusive settings. But premature limitation of service time and premature reliance on group instruction are counterproductive strategies that should be ended.

Redesign educational services for young school-age children, that is, children from five through seven, who have autism. For those children who have not yet acquired language, instruction should be focused on establishing systems of communication. If the child is not demonstrating progress in developing functional speech, an alternative mode of communication should be taught, while speech instruction continues. This process requires blocks of one-to-one instructional time for students with teachers and/or speech-language therapists. A pre-kindergarten or kindergarten curriculum implemented primarily through group instruction does not constitute an adequate or appropriate instructional program for autistic children without functional language.

Instructional support is also needed in another vital area—namely communicating, playing, and learning with typical children. A variety of strategies have been devised to develop such skills and to help children benefit from experiences in inclusive settings. At present, children with autism do not have sufficient opportunities for carefully planned, graduated, and adequately supported participation in mainstream classes. This needs to change.

Make the use of augmentative and alternative means of communication an integral part of the life of older students who do not have functional speech or whose speech is too limited to allow them to express their ideas fully. In one program for autistic students of high school age, I watched and listened to a small group discussion of a science topic being conducted in the school library. A boy of about sixteen did not participate, although he appeared to be alert to what was going on. I asked the program administrator about him and was told that although he was bright and could write, he didn't speak. No pad, pen or pencil, typewriter, computer, or special communication device was in sight in the area where the discussion was taking place. Nor did the teacher request any communication from that student or address any questions or comments to him. This was not an isolated example of students without adequate support for communication, either in that particular school or in others.

A substantial number of autistic individuals do not acquire functional speech. In addition to common tools for writing, a variety of special communication devices are available today for individuals of different ages and achievement levels. There is no excuse for any individual in any setting to be without an effective means of communication. We have been lax about ensuring that this does not occur; and we have not been vigorous enough in encouraging and supporting communication through an alternative mode when this is the only viable means of establishing communication. Professional passivity in this context fosters continued isolation and dependence on the part of the autistic individual.

Provide more intensive preparation for teachers in the strategies and skills needed to work productively with young children who have autism or other pervasive developmental disorders. While there are some commonalities in the learning needs of typical students or students with mild disabilities and autistic children, there are also many differences. It is not realistic to expect every teacher to have the skill to work with autistic children, but it is reasonable to expect special education teachers and early childhood teachers to have an understanding of the special learning difficulties and needs of young children with pervasive developmental disabilities. At the present time this is often not the case.

In-service training is one mechanism for supplementing what teachers have learned in their college-based teacher education programs. It is a potentially valuable mechanism for developing better skills in teachers who work with autistic students. More schools and school systems need to take advantage of this opportunity by utilizing personnel from programs with demonstrated effectiveness in educating autistic students to provide in-service training and consultation to teachers and supervisors who are not skilled at working with this student population.

In-service training of college-based teacher educators is essential too. When parents began calling me in late 1993, seeking students to work in Lovaas-type in-home programs, I knew little about the most recent developments in the behavioral treatment of autistic children; and I was a teacher educator who had both experience and serious interest in the education of autistic children. What about the others?

We have been focusing on children with autism; but these children become adolescents and young adults with autism, and most of them continue to need special services or supports, even when they do well in most areas of academic work. It would take another book to outline the kinds of educational assistance of benefit to older children, adolescents, and young adults. Without taking on this task, I will describe one aspect of such services. Educational planning for adolescents and young adults should revolve about the conceptualization of adult life for the particular individual in focus. And how do we formulate this conceptualization, readers may ask. Fortunately, some very thoughtful and skilled professionals have been grappling with that question for over a decade.

"Person-centered planning" is a term used to describe strategies to identify and pursue what a person with a disability wants and needs. Other names associated with this process are "Life Style Planning" and "Personal Futures Planning" (Kincaid 1996, 440). The process starts with the coming together of everyone who is significant in the life of the individual (along with that person himself or herself), with each person participating by sharing information about the individual's functioning and a vision for the individual's future. The outcome of this exploration is a picture of the overall themes that impact on the person's life, and the outcomes to be sought. Barriers to achieving those outcomes, and strategies for dealing with these barriers, are also examined. This process differs from more common types of planning in that it does not limit itself to one part of the person's life; the planning group is not limited to paid professionals and parents; and the current restrictions of service systems are not viewed as insurmountable obstacles that should narrow the options being considered for the life envisioned.

Person-centered planning was designed primarily for persons with severe disabilities who could not easily define or communicate what they wanted or needed. Yet such planning is equally relevant for older autistic students who are referred to as "high functioning" but who nonetheless may not have a good sense of their futures as adults or ways to get where they want to go.

"Getting a life" is the overall theme and purpose of person-centered planning, and that's what happened to Jay Turnbull. Ann Turnbull, Jay's mother and a highly respected special educator, was a keynote speaker at the national conference of the Autism Society of America in 1995. The theme of her presentation was creating enviable lives for individuals with autism. Jay's family was unwilling to accept his life as it had become in young adulthood. And Jay communicated to them by his actions—head banging, hitting, choking, hair pulling, and refusal to get up in the morning—that his life was not the life that he wanted. The lifestyle that Jay Turnbull's family envisioned for him, and believed Jay too wanted, was one of living, working, and participating in the community; not working in a large group of other people with severe disabilities at assembly-line packaging tasks, living with other people with severe disabilities, traveling in segregated groups, and interacting almost exclusively with other people with severe disabilities in a sheltered workshop or group home. Jay's family made a commitment to do everything necessary to help make Jay's envisioned life a reality.

The strategies the Turnbulls used to help Jay achieve a better life combined a person-centered planning process with positive behavioral supports. The planning process itself—the motivation, enthusiasm, and problem solving it generated—along with the intensive, comprehensive support system that developed in the planning process, enabled Jay Turnbull, after a long and difficult period (which Ann Turnbull identified as about six years), to achieve the lifestyle envisioned for him. The criterion used to evaluate success was Jay's changed behavior: his greater independence, his reliable work as a clerical aide, his contacts and activities in the community, and the striking decrease in the challenging behaviors that he had exhibited.

Jim Sinclair is a highly intelligent, well educated adult, editor of the newsletter *Our Voice*, and writer of a poem included in chapter 2 of this book. Yet Jim Sinclair has gone through long periods of unemployment. Moreover, a substantial number of other intelligent and well-educated adults with autism have had similar experiences. No person-centered planning process or personalized support system was available when Jim Sinclair and other autistic adults like him needed it. Such a process might have helped make their lives considerably more satisfying and productive. We can't afford to allow these wasted opportunities to continue.

We do not yet know enough to enable most individuals with autism to attain enviable lives. Nor can most families create the mixture of supports also needed to attain such an outcome. But we have learned enough in recent years to help more and more individuals with autism go on to productive and satisfying lives.

We "typicals" carefully delineate the deficiencies of people with autism in being able to take the point of view of others, but can we, ourselves, switch lenses and look at the world from the perspective of "autistics"? The Autism Network International (ANI) is a self-advocacy association of adults with autism, and from time to time it publishes a newsletter, *Our Voice*, composed largely of contributions from its members. The newsletter's dominant themes are the struggle involved in functioning, the discomfort and distress of being with typical people, the battle to have pride in one's self as an autistic person, and the pleasure of relating to other people with autism.

There is much in *Our Voice* to make us question current conceptualizations of autism. True, the contributors to this newsletter represent only a small segment of the autistic population, but they are not excluded from the generalizations about people with autism. Are people with autism unable to take the point of view of others or do they have great difficulty with the process because the "others" in question are "typicals"? Do autistic individuals have this problem when the "other" is another person with autism? Are typical people any better at taking the viewpoint of people with autism than autistic people are in taking that of people with typical development? Researchers might examine these questions. To the best of my knowledge no one has.

Can people with autism have friendships and adult love relationships? Many adults with autism haven't had either; and Temple Grandin's own reports about lack of friendships, dates, flirtations, boyfriends, or romantic feelings support the notion that people with autism don't have such feelings and can't have such relationships. But that is certainly not true of all people with autism. Donna Williams and Georgiana Stehli have married, as have other adults with autism who are not as well known. Some autistic adults very much want to have girlfriends or boyfriends and love relationships, and they actively pursue those possibilities. Paul McDonnell reported that after his second year of high school his interest in girls began with a vengeance, and he began searching almost desperately for a girlfriend.

Temple Grandin concludes from her observations that "marriages work out best when two people with autism marry or when a person with autism marries . . . [an] eccentric spouse . . . [so that] their intellects work on a similar wavelength" (1995, 133). Sacks, in describing a married couple in which both people had Asperger's syndrome, writes: "They recognized their own autism, and they had recognized each other's, at college, with a sense of such affinity and delight that it was inevitable they would marry. 'It was as if we had known each other for a million years,'" the wife remarked (1995, 276). Yet to the best of my knowledge no one has studied marriages involving adults with autism, including marriages of two people with autism as well as "mixed marriages" of an autistic adult and a "typical." One such mixed couple, writing in *Our Voice*, reported that each of them had to work very hard at understanding the other, and each of them experienced culture shock. Yet what they also described was a close bond between them. The autistic husband felt very lucky to have found a partner like his wife, and the nonautistic wife reported that "for every time his autism drives me absolutely crazy, there are 4 or 5 times that it simply delights me" (Wiebe and Wiebe n.d., 15).

Putting aside for the moment the deficiencies and dysfunctions that occupy most of the attention of researchers and clinicians, we can cheer at some of the strengths of people with autism. One such characteristic is the continued learning throughout adulthood of some individuals with autism. Temple Grandin has grown greatly during her adult years—in self-awareness, in social skills, and in interpersonal relationships. She is beginning to talk about her friends, and to enjoy the company of the few to whom she gives that designation.

In an article in *Our Voice*, Jean-Paul Bovee writes that the highlight of an annual conference of the Autism Society of America was meeting with his friends from ANI. Another newsletter contributor writes about an autistic friend who sang to her and how much that meant. What they have together, these friends, is that they can be themselves with one another, without being concerned about how their behavior looks in the world of typicals and without being asked to change.

Donna Williams has been a contributor to *Our Voice*, and one topic her contributions addressed is her attitude toward her own autism. The self-advocacy movement has reached the members of this network, and some questioned Donna Williams's writings on this subject. She responded: "Autism is sometimes my sanctuary and sometimes my prison. When it imprisons me, I am at war with it. . . . The point is, not to fight autism per se, but to fight it *only for the right reasons.* . . . I will fight confinement wherever I find it" (Williams n.d., 6, 8).

Temple Grandin, who has found ways of circumventing many of the imprisoning aspects of her autism, tells us, "I think lots of times there are things missing from my life." But, she also states, "if I could snap my fingers and be nonautistic, I would not—because then I wouldn't be me" (Sacks 1995, 286, 291).

Dreams live on. William and Barbara Christopher, parents of twenty-year-old Ned, still have wishful dreams of their son being free of the confusion and pain that have marked much of his life. In these dreams Ned is married, has a good job, and makes his own decisions. But the only sound insurance for their son and others like him, the Christophers conclude, is a society that comes to value every person, irrespective of what he or she can do.

appendix a Diagnostic Criteria
for Autistic Disorder

Reprinted with permission from the *Diagnostic and Statistical Manual of Mental Disorders*, 4th ed. (Washington, D.C.: American Psychiatric Association, 1994).

A. A total of six (or more) items from (1), (2), and (3), with at least two from (1), and one each from (2) and (3).

(1) qualitative impairment in social interaction, as manifested by at least two of the following:

(a) marked impairment in the use of multiple nonverbal behaviors such as eye-to-eye gaze, facial expression, body postures, and gestures to regulate social interaction

(b) failure to develop peer relationships appropriate to developmental level

(c) a lack of spontaneous seeking to share enjoyment, interests, or achievements with other people (e.g., by a lack of showing, bringing, or pointing out objects of interest)

(d) lack of social or emotional reciprocity

187

(2) qualitative impairments in communication as manifested by at least one of the following:

    (a) delay in, or total lack of, the development of spoken language (not accompanied by an attempt to compensate through alternative modes of communication such as gesture or mime)

    (b) in individuals with adequate speech, marked impairment in the ability to initiate or sustain a conversation with others

    (c) stereotyped and repetitive use of language or idiosyncratic language

    (d) lack of varied, spontaneous make-believe play or social imitative play appropriate to developmental level

(3) restricted repetitive and stereotyped patterns of behavior, interests, and activities, as manifested by at least one of the following:

    (a) encompassing preoccupation with one or more stereotyped and restricted patterns of interest that is abnormal either in intensity or focus

    (b) apparently inflexible adherence to specific, nonfunctional routines or rituals

    (c) stereotyped and repetitive motor mannerisms (e.g., hand or finger flapping or twisting, or complex whole-body movements)

    (d) persistent preoccupation with parts of objects

B. Delays or abnormal functioning in at least one of the following areas, with onset prior to 3 years: (1) social interaction, (2) language as used in social communication, or (3) symbolic or imaginative play.

C. The disturbance is not better accounted for by Rett's Disorder or Childhood Disintegrative Disorder.

appendix b Resources

GENERAL INFORMATION RESOURCES

Please note that this list of resources is not meant to be exhaustive. It provides some major sources of information, referral, and training for parents and professionals who don't know where to get started. More comprehensive lists of resources have been compiled by the Autism Society of America and other organizations.

Autism Society of America
7910 Woodmont Avenue, Suite 300
Bethesda, MD 20814–3067
Telephone: 800-3-AUTISM
Web Site: www.autism-society.org
Fax: (301) 657-0869

The Autism Society of America is a broad-based national organization that provides a variety of types of information and referral services to the public—and an excellent starting point for learning more about autism. Information packages

189

are available at the ASA web site. ASA publishes a newsletter four times a year. The Autism Society of America has over 200 chapters. It will furnish information about the chapter closest to the person making an inquiry. (The annual membership fee for an individual is $25.)

Autism Research Institute
4182 Adams Avenue
San Diego, CA 92116
Telephone: (619) 281-7165
Web Site: www.autism.com/ari

The Autism Research Institute is concerned with research into methods of treating autism. One of its functions is to provide information to parents and professionals on the latest findings in this area. This institute is an excellent source of information on alternative treatment methods. ARI publishes a quarterly newsletter, the *Autism Research Review International,* and it sells information packs and books relevant to the treatment of autism.

National Information Center for Children and Youth with Disabilities (NICHCY)
P.O. Box 1492
Washington, DC 20013
Telephone: (800) 695-0285
Web Site: www.nichcy.org

This center provides free information to parents and professionals about resources for children with various types of disabilities, including autism.

SPECIALIZED INFORMATION RESOURCES

Asperger Syndrome Coalition of the U.S. (ASC-U.S.)
(formerly known as Aspen of America)
P.O. Box 49267
Jacksonville Beach, FL 32240
Telephone: (904) 745-6741
Web Site: www.asperger.org

The Asperger Syndrome Coalition of the U.S. is a national volunteer, not-for-profit organization committed to efforts that enable individuals with Asperger syndrome and related disorders to realize their potential.

CAN (Cure Autism NOW)
5225 Wilshire Blvd., Suite 503
Los Angeles, CA 90036
Telephone: (213) 549-0500
Fax: (213) 549-0547
Web Site: www.canfoundation.org

This parent-founded organization funds research on biological treatments for autism. CAN's internet web page is for parents and researchers who share the vision of a cure for autism. This web site will include a database of abstracts of all research on autism from 1966 to the present.

Clinic for the Behavioral Treatment of Children
(O. Ivar Lovaas, Director)
Department of Psychology
1282A Franz Hall, P.O. Box 951563
University of California
Los Angeles, CA 90095-1563
Telephone: (310) 825-2319

Lovaas Institute for Early Intervention (LIFE)
2566 Overland Ave.
Suite #530
Los Angeles, CA 90064
Telephone: (310) 840-5983
e-mail: info@lovaas.com
Web Site: www.lovaas.com

The Clinic for the Behavioral Treatment of Children conducts research on autism under the direction of Ivar Lovaas. The Lovaas Institute for Early Intervention (LIFE) provides workshops for starting in-home programs as well as consultation and services in the local area. Either center above will provide information about services.

Division TEACCH
The Division for Treatment and Education
of Autistic and Related Communication Handicapped Children
University of North Carolina, Chapel Hill
School of Medicine
310 Medical School, Wing E, CB 7180
Chapel Hill, NC 27599-7180

Telephone: (919) 966-2174
e-mail: teacch@unc.edu
Web Site: www.unc.edu/depts/teacch/teacch.htm

Division TEACCH offers a variety of training workshops for teachers and other professionals working with children, adolescents, and adults with autism, utilizing the approach developed by this system.

The Family Connection
Beach Center on Families and Disability
3111 Haworth Hall
University of Kansas
Lawrence, KS 66045
Telephone: (800) 854-4938
e-mail: Family@dole.lsi.ukans.edu
Web Site: www.lsi.ukans.edu/beach/beachhp.htm

The Family Connection of the Beach Center on Families and Disabilities focuses on challenging behavior. Parents who contact this resource will be put in touch with a state training team on positive behavioral supports if they reside in any of the 20 states that have such teams. Otherwise, parents will be helped to network with other parents and contact professionals in their area who are skilled in the use of positive behavioral supports with individuals who have challenging behavior.

Stanley I. Greenspan, M.D.
7201 Glenbrook Road
Bethesda, MD 20814
Telephone: (301) 657-2348

Dr. Greenspan is available for four-session evaluations of young children with developmental disorders, after which he recommends a treatment program. (For persons who do not live in or near Maryland, he will do the four sessions in one day.) The treatment recommended often includes speech therapy, occupational therapy with a sensory integration focus, interactive play therapy, an interactive school program that uses Dr. Greenspan's "floor time" model as its core, and extension of the floor-time principles to the home.

Pyramid Educational Consultants
226 West Park Place, Suite #1
Newark, DE 19711
Telephone: (888) 732-7462
e-mail: pyramid@pecs.com
Web Site: www.pecs.com

This company, headed by Andrew S. Bondy and Lori Frost, sells the PECS (Picture Exchange Communication System) manual and presents workshops for parents and professionals on its use.

PARENT GROUPS

Numerous local parent groups have sprung up during the 1990s to advocate early, intensive treatment of young children with autism. As there is no directory that includes all of these groups, interested parents should ask professionals and other parents at evaluation and treatment centers about the availability of parent groups in their area. Other sources of information are the Autism Society of America (national and state chapters), the National Information Center for Children and Youth with Disabilities, the Asperger Syndrome Coalition of the U.S., and FEAT. FEAT, which stands for Families for Early Autism Treatment, is a parent-run, nonprofit, volunteer network that has local organizations in several states and also publishes an online newsletter. Its web site is www.feat.org.

INTERNET

There are numerous web sites that have information on or related to autism. It is important to know the source of the information provided and to evaluate the quality of that information. The National Alliance for Autism Research (NAAR) publishes information on a variety of subjects related to autism, particularly medical research. That web site is www.naar.org. A web site that provides a large amount of information as well as links is Autism Resources at www.autism-info.com.

References

American Psychiatric Association. 1994. *Diagnostic and statistical manual of mental disorders.* 4th ed. Washington, D.C.: American Psychiatric Association.

Anderson, Stephen R., Debra L. Avery, Ellette K. DiPietro, Glynnis L. Edwards, and Walter P. Christian. 1987. Intensive home-based early intervention with autistic children. *Education and Treatment of Children* 10:352–66.

Baron-Cohen, Simon. 1995. *Mindblindness: An essay on autism and theory of mind.* Cambridge, Mass.: MIT Press.

Baron-Cohen, Simon, Antony Cox, Gillian Baird, John Swettenham, Natasha Nightingale, Kate Morgan, Auriol Drew, and Tony Charman. 1996. Psychological markers in the detection of autism in infancy in a large population. *British Journal of Psychiatry* 168:158–63.

Baron-Cohen, Simon, and Patricia Howlin. 1993. The theory of mind deficit in autism: Some questions for teaching and diagnosis. In *Understanding other minds: Perspectives from autism,* ed. Simon Baron-Cohen, Helen Tager-Flusberg, and Donald J. Cohen, 466–80. New York: Oxford University Press.

Barron, Judy, and Sean Barron. 1992. *There's a boy in here.* New York: Avon.

Bauman, Margaret L. 1996. Brief report: Neuroanatomic observations of the brain in pervasive developmental disorders. *Journal of Autism and Developmental Disorders* 26:199–203.

Bauman, Margaret L., and Thomas L. Kemper. 1994. Neuroanatomic observations of the brain in autism. In *The neurobiology of autism*, ed. Margaret L. Bauman and Thomas L. Kemper, 119–45. Baltimore: Johns Hopkins University Press.

Bemporad, Jules R. 1979. Adult recollections of a formerly autistic child. *Journal of Autism and Developmental Disorders* 9:179–97.

Bettison, Sue. 1996. The long-term effects of auditory training on children with autism. *Journal of Autism and Developmental Disorders* 26:361–74.

Biklen, Douglas. 1992. Autism orthodoxy versus free speech: A reply to Cummins and Prior. *Harvard Educational Review* 62:242–56.

Birnbrauer, Jay S., and David J. Leach. 1993. The Murdoch early intervention program after 2 years. *Behaviour Change* 10:63–74.

Bondy, Andrew S., and Lori A. Frost. 1994. The Delaware autistic program. In *Preschool education programs for children with autism*, ed. Sandra L. Harris and Jan S. Handleman, 37–54. Austin, Tex.: PRO-ED.

Bovee, Jean-Paul. 1995. Jean-Paul. *Advocate* 27 (March–April): 6–7.

Brantlinger, Ellen A., Susan M. Klein, and Samuel L. Guskin. 1994. *Fighting for Darla: The case study of a pregnant adolescent with autism, challenges for family care and professional responsibility.* New York: Teachers College Press.

Bruner, Jerome, and Carol Feldman. 1993. Theories of mind and the problem of autism. In *Understanding other minds: Perspectives from autism*, ed. Simon Baron-Cohen, Helen Tager-Flusberg, and Donald J. Cohen, 267–91. New York: Oxford University Press.

Callahan, Mary. 1987. *Fighting for Tony.* New York: Simon and Schuster.

Carpenter, Anne. 1992. Autistic adulthood: A challenging journey. In *High-functioning individuals with autism*, ed. Eric Schopler and Gary B. Mesibov, 289–294. New York: Plenum.

Cesaroni, Laura, and Malcolm Garber. 1991. Exploring the experience of autism through firsthand accounts. *Journal of Autism and Developmental Disorders* 21:303–13.

Christopher, William, and Barbara Christopher. 1989. *Mixed blessings.* Nashville, Tenn.: Abingdon.

Church, Catherine C., and James Coplan. 1995. The high-functioning autistic experience: Birth to preteen years. *Journal of Pediatric Health Care* 9:22–29.

Courchesne, Eric, Alan J. Lincoln, Jeanne P. Townsend, Hector E. James, Natacha A. Akshoomoff, Osamu Saitoh, Rachel Yeung-Courchesne, Brian Egaas, Gary A. Press, Richard H. Haas, James W. Murakami, and Laura Schreibman. 1994. A new finding: Impairment in shifting attention in autistic and cerebellar patients. In *Atypical cognitive deficits in developmental disorders: Implications for brain function*, ed. Sarah H. Broman and Jordan Grafman, 101–37. Hillsdale, N.J.: Erlbaum.

Dawson, Geraldine. 1991. A psychobiological perspective on the early socioemotional development of children with autism. In *Rochester symposium on developmental psychopathology: Models and integrations*, ed. Dante Cicchetti and Sheree I. Toth, 3:207–34. Rochester, N.Y.: University of Rochester Press.

DeMyer, Marian K., Sandra Barton, William E. DeMyer, James A. Norton, John Allen, and Robert Steele. 1973. Prognosis in autism: A follow-up study. *Journal of Autism and Childhood Schizophrenia* 3:199–246.

Denckla, Martha. 1996. Brain mechanisms. *Journal of Autism and Developmental Disorders* 26:134–40.

DePaolo, Steffie. 1995. The ups and downs of silence. *Advocate* 27 (May–June): 9.

Department of Health and Human Services, National Institutes of Health. 1995. *The human genome project: From maps to medicine*. NIH Publication no. 95–3897. Bethesda, Md.: National Institutes of Health.

Dewey, Margaret. 1991. Living with Asperger's syndrome. In *Autism and Asperger syndrome*, ed. Uta Frith, 184–206. New York: Cambridge University Press.

Donnellan, Anne M., and Martha R. Leary. 1995. *Movement differences and diversity in autism/mental retardation: Appreciating and accommodating people with communication and behavior challenges*. Madison, Wis.: DRI Press.

Donnelly, Julia A. 1994. Excerpts from the young adults with autism panel: Speaking for ourselves, ASA 1994 Las Vegas. *Advocate* 26 (November–December): 7.

Donovan, William J. 1971. My experiences as an autistic child. In *Conference and annual meeting of the National Society for Autistic Children, San Francisco, June 24–27, 1970*, ed. Clara C. Park, 99–103. Public Health Services Publication no. 2164. Rockville, Md.: National Institutes of Mental Health.

Eaves, Linda C., and Helena H. Ho. 1996. Brief report: Stability and change in cognitive and behavioral characteristics of autism through childhood. *Journal of Autism and Developmental Disorders* 26:557–69.

Eisenberg, Leon, and Leo Kanner. 1956. Childhood schizophrenia: Symposium, 1955–56. Early infantile autism, 1943–55. *American Journal of Orthopsychiatry* 26:556–66.

Gajzago, Christine, and Margot Prior. 1974. Two cases of "recovery" in Kanner syndrome. *Archives of General Psychiatry* 31:264–68.

Gilbert, K. 1995. Preserving reality of autism. *Advocate* 27 (July–August): 4.

Gillberg, Christopher. 1991. Outcome in autism and autistic-like conditions. *Journal of the Academy of Child and Adolescent Psychiatry* 30:375–82.

Gilpin, R. Wayne. 1993. *Laughing and loving with autism—a collection of "real life" warm and humorous stories.* Arlington, Tex.: Future Horizons.

———. 1994. *More laughing and loving with autism—a collection of "real life" warm and humorous stories.* Arlington, Tex.: Future Horizons.

Gollan, Kathy. 1996. The Health Report: Autism—a special report by Kathy Gollan. Sydney, Australia: Radio National, July 29.

Goodwin, Mary S., and T. Campbell Goodwin. 1969. In a dark mirror. *Mental Hygiene* 53:550–63.

Grandin, Temple. 1992. An inside view of autism. In *High-functioning individuals with autism,* ed. Eric Schopler and Gary B. Mesibov, 105–26. New York: Plenum.

———. 1995. How people with autism think. In *Learning and cognition in autism,* ed. Eric Schopler and Gary B. Mesibov, 137–56. New York: Plenum.

Grandin, Temple, and Margaret M. Scariano. 1986. *Emergence: Labeled autistic.* Novato, Calif.: Arena.

Green, Gina. 1996. Evaluating claims about treatments for autism. In *Behavioral intervention for young children with autism,* ed. Catherine Maurice, Gina Green, and Stephen C. Luce, 15–28. Austin, Tex.: PRO-ED.

Greenfeld, Josh. 1972. *A child called Noah: A family journey.* New York: Holt, Rinehart and Winston.

———. 1978. *A place for Noah.* New York: Harcourt Brace Jovanovich.

Greenspan, Stanley I. 1992a. *Infancy and early childhood: The practice of clinical assessment and intervention with emotional and developmental challenges.* Madison, Ct.: International Universities Press.

———. 1992b. Reconsidering the diagnosis and treatment of very young children with autistic spectrum or pervasive developmental disorder. *Zero to Three* 13, no. 2:1–9.

———. 1997. *Developmentally based psychotherapy.* Madison, Ct.: International Universities Press.

Happe, Francesca. 1991. The autobiographical writings of three Asperger syndrome adults: Problems of interpretation and implications for theory. In *Autism and Asperger syndrome,* ed. Uta Frith, 207–42. New York: Cambridge University Press.

Harris, Sandra L. 1994. *Siblings of children with autism: A guide for families.* Bethesda, Md.: Woodbine House.

Hart, Charles. 1989. *Without reason: A family copes with two generations of autism.* New York: Harper and Row.

Huff, Ronald C. 1996. Community-based early intervention for children with autism. In *Behavioral intervention for young children with autism: A manual for parents and professionals,* ed. Catherine Maurice, Gina Green, and Stephen C. Luce, 251–66. Austin, Tex.: PRO-ED.

Hundley, Joan M. 1971. *The small outsider: The story of an autistic child.* New York: St. Martin's Press.

Hurlburt, Russell T., Francesca Happe, and Uta Frith. 1994. Sampling the form of inner experience in three adults with Asperger syndrome. *Psychological Medicine* 24:385–95.

Interview with Ivar Lovaas. 1994. *Advocate* 26 (November–December): 19–23.

An interview with Ruth Christ Sullivan. 1995. *Advocate* 27 (November–December): 9–15.

Isaiah. 1995. A brother's view. *Advocate* 27 (September–October): 7.

Jacobson, John W., James A. Mulick, and Allen A. Schwartz. 1995. A history of facilitated communication: Science, pseudoscience, and antiscience. *American Psychologist* 50:750–65.

Jasinski, Jean. 1995. Jason. In *Dancing in the rain: Stories of exceptional progress by parents of children with special needs,* ed. Annabel Stehli, 1–20. Westport, Conn.: The Georgiana Organization.

Johnson, Carol, and Julia Crowder. 1994. *Autism: From tragedy to triumph.* Boston: Brandon Books.

Kanner, Leo. 1973. *Childhood psychosis: Initial studies and new insights.* Washington, D.C.: Winston.

Kaufman, Barry N. 1976. *Son rise.* New York: Warner Books.

———. 1994. *Son rise: The miracle continues.* Tiburon, Calif.: Kramer.

Kiebala, Eileen S. 1995. Patrick. *Advocate* 27 (July–August): 10–11.

Kincaid, Don. 1996. Person-centered planning. In *Positive behavioral support: Including people with difficult behavior in the community,* ed. Lynn K. Koegel, Robert L. Koegel, and Glen Dunlap, 439–63. Baltimore, Md.: Paul Brookes.

Klin, Ami, and Fred R. Volkmar. 1995. *Asperger syndrome: Some guidelines for assessment, diagnosis, and intervention.* Pittsburgh, Pa.: Learning Disabilities Association of America.

Koegel, Robert L., William D. Frea, and Alan V. Surratt. 1994. Self-management of problematic social behavior. In *Behavioral issues in autism,* ed. Eric Schopler and Gary B. Mesibov, 81–97. New York: Plenum.

Koegel, Robert L., and Lynn K. Koegel, eds. 1995. *Teaching children with autism: Strategies for initiating positive interactions and improving learning opportunities.* Baltimore, Md.: Paul Brookes.

Koplow, Lesley, Suzanne Abrams, Judy Ferber, and Beverly Dennis. 1996. Helping children with pervasive developmental disorders. In *Unsmiling faces: How preschools can heal,* ed. Lesley Koplow, 181–201. New York: Teachers College Press.

Leakey, Richard. 1994. *The origin of humankind.* New York: Basic Books.

Lewis, Mark H., John P. Gluck, James W. Bodfish, Alan J. Beauchamp, and Richard B. Mailman. 1996. Neurobiological basis of stereotyped movement disorder. In *Stereotyped movements: Brain and behavior relationships,* ed. Robert L. Sprague and Karl M. Newell, 37–67. Washington, D.C.: American Psychological Association.

Lord, Catherine. 1995. Follow-up of two-year-olds referred for possible autism. *Journal of Child Psychology and Psychiatry* 36:1365–82.

Lord, Catherine, and Michael Rutter. 1994. Autism and pervasive developmental disorders. In *Child and adolescent psychiatry: Modern approaches,* ed. Michael Rutter, Eric Taylor, and Lionel Hersov. 3d ed. Oxford: Blackwell Scientific Publications.

Lord, Catherine, and Eric Schopler. 1989a. The role of age at assessment, developmental level, and test in the stability of intelligence scores in young autistic children. *Journal of Autism and Developmental Disorders* 19:483–99.

———. 1989b. Stability of assessment results of autistic and non-autistic language-impaired children from preschool years to early school age. *Journal of Child Psychology and Psychiatry* 30:575–90.

———. 1994. TEACCH services for preschool children. In *Preschool programs for children with autism,* ed. Sandra L. Harris and Jan S. Handleman, 87–106. Austin, Tex.: PRO-ED.

Lotter, Victor. 1978. Follow-up studies. In *Autism: A reappraisal of concepts and treatment,* ed. Michael Rutter and Eric Schopler, 475–95. New York: Plenum.

Lovaas, O. Ivar. 1981. *Teaching developmentally disabled children: The ME book.* Austin, Tex.: PRO-ED.

———. 1987. Behavioral treatment and normal educational and intellectual functioning in young autistic children. *Journal of Consulting and Clinical Psychology* 55:3–9.

———. 1996. The UCLA young autism model of service delivery. In *Behavioral intervention for young children with autism: A manual for parents and professionals,* ed. Catherine Maurice, Gina Green, and Stephen C. Luce, 241–48. Austin, Tex.: PRO-ED.

Lovaas, O. Ivar, and Gregory Buch. 1997. Intensive behavioral intervention with young children with autism. In *Prevention and treatment of severe behavior problems: Models and method in developmental disabilities,* ed. Nirbhay N. Singh, 61–86. Pacific Grove, Calif.: Brooks/Cole.

Makarushka, M. 1991. The words they can't say. *New York Times Magazine,* October 6, 32–33, 36, 70.

Maurice, Catherine. 1993. *Let me hear your voice: A family's triumph over autism.* New York: Fawcett Columbine.

Maurice, Catherine, Gina Green, and Stephen C. Luce, eds. 1996. *Behavioral intervention for young children with autism: A manual for parents and professionals.* Austin, Tex.: PRO-ED.

McDonnell, Jane T. 1993. *News from the border: A mother's memoir of her autistic son.* New York: Ticknor and Fields.

McEachin, John J., Tristram Smith, and O. Ivar Lovaas. 1993. Long-term outcome for children with autism who received early intensive behavioral treatment. *American Journal on Mental Retardation* 97:359–72.

McKean, Thomas A. 1994. *Soon will come the light: A view from inside the autism puzzle.* Arlington, Tex.: Future Education.

Miller, Arnold, and Ellen Eller-Miller. 1989. *From ritual to repertoire: A cognitive-developmental systems approach with behavior-disordered children.* New York: Wiley.

Mirenda, Patricia L., and Anne M. Donnellan. 1987. Issues in curriculum development. In *Handbook of autism and pervasive developmental disorders,* ed. Donald J. Cohen, Anne M. Donnellan, and Rhea Paul, 211–26. New York: John Wiley.

Morphett, Lurline. 1986. *Face to face.* South Australia: Education Department of South Australia.

Mundy, Peter. 1993. Normal versus high-functioning status in children with autism. *American Journal on Mental Retardation* 97:381–84.

Nickelsen, Fallon. 1996. Erik. *Advocate* 28 (March–April): 4.

Oppenheim, Rosalind C. 1974. *Effective teaching methods for autistic children.* Springfield, Ill.: Charles C. Thomas.

Park, Clara Claiborne. 1982. *The siege: The first eight years of an autistic child, with an epilogue, fifteen years later.* Boston: Little, Brown.

———. 1986. Social growth in autism: A parent's perspective. In *Social behavior in autism,* ed. Eric Schopler and Gary B. Mesibov, 81–99. New York: Plenum.

———, ed. 1971. *Conference and annual meeting of the National Society for Autistic Children, San Francisco, June 24–27, 1970.* Public Health Services Publication no. 2164. Rockville, Md.: National Institute of Mental Health.

Pfeiffer, Steven I., Jennifer Norton, Laura Nelson, and Susan Shott. 1995. Efficacy of vitamin B6 and magnesium in the treatment of autism: A methodological review and summary of outcomes. *Journal of Autism and Developmental Disorders* 25:481–93.

Pinney, Rachel, and Mimi Schlachter. 1983. *Bobby: Breakthrough of a special child.* New York: St. Martin's/Marek.

Plioplys, Audrius V. 1994. Autism: Electroencephalogram abnormalities and clinical improvement with valproic acid. *Archives of Pediatrics and Adolescent Medicine* 148:220–22.

Prizant, Barry M., and Amy M. Wetherby. 1989. Providing services to children with autism ages 0–2 and their families. *Focus on Autistic Behavior* 4, no. 2:1–16.

Rapin, Isabelle. 1994. Introduction and overview. In *The neurobiology of autism,* ed. Margaret L. Bauman and Thomas L. Kemper, 1–17. Baltimore, Md.: Johns Hopkins University.

Rapoport, Judith L. 1989. *The boy who couldn't stop washing: The experience and treatment of obsessive-compulsive disorder.* New York: New American Library.

Rimland, Bernard. 1964. *Infantile autism: The syndrome and its implications for a neural theory of behavior.* New York: Appleton-Century-Crofts.

Rimland, Bernard, and Stephen M. Edelson. 1994. The effects of auditory integration training on autism. *American Journal of Speech-Language Pathology* 3:16–24.

Rogers, Sally J. 1996a. Brief report: Early intervention in autism. *Journal of Autism and Developmental Disorders* 26:243–46.

————. 1996b. Teaching imitation and symbolic play. In *The child with special needs preconference: Autism: State of the art informed by state of the science,* 133–43. Conference sponsored by Contemporary Forums, May, Washington, D.C.

Rutter, Michael. 1983. Cognitive deficits in the pathogenesis of autism. *Journal of Child Psychology and Psychiatry* 24:513–31.

Sacks, Oliver. 1995. *An anthropologist on Mars: Seven paradoxical tales.* New York: Knopf.

Schloss, Hadassah M. 1995. Reality reminder [Letters to the Advocate]. *Advocate* 27 (March–April): 5.

Schulze, Craig B. 1993. *When snow turns to rain: One family's struggle to solve the riddle of autism.* Rockville, Md.: Woodbine House.

Sinclair, J. 1992. Bridging the gaps: An inside-out view of autism. In *High-functioning individuals with autism,* ed. Eric Schopler and Gary B. Mesibov, 294–302. New York: Plenum.

Strain, Phillip S., Frank W. Kohler, and Howard Goldstein. 1996. Learning experiences . . . an alternative program: Peer mediated interventions for young children with autism. In *Child and adolescent disorders: Empirically based strategies for clinical practice,* ed. Euthymia D. Hibbs and Peter S. Jensen, 573–87. Washington, D.C.: American Psychological Association.

Swanson, Joan, and Curt Sytsma. 1995. *Judicial and ALJ interpretations of the FAPE requirement for pre-school children with autism: A synthesis of recent developments.* Des Moines: Iowa Protection and Advocacy Services.

Szatmari, Peter, Giampierro Bartolucci, R. Bremner, S. Bond, and S. Rich. 1989. A follow-up study of high-functioning autistic children. *Journal of Autism and Developmental Disorders* 19:213–25.

Taylor, Bridget A., and Kelly A. McDonough. 1996. Selecting teaching programs. In *Behavioral intervention for young children with autism,* ed. Catherine Maurice, Gina Green, and Stephen C. Luce, 63–177. Austin, Tex.: PRO-ED.

Teitelbaum, Philip, Ralph G. Maurer, Joshua Fryman, Osnat B. Teitelbaum, Joel Vilensky, and Margaret P. Creedon. 1996. Dimensions of disintegration in the stereotyped locomotion characteristic of Parkinsonism and autism. In *Stereotyped movements: Brain and behavior relationships,* ed. Robert L. Sprague and Karl M. Newell, 167–93. Washington, D.C.: American Psychological Association.

Volkmar, Fred R. 1993. Autism and the pervasive developmental disorders. In *Handbook of infant mental health,* ed. Charles H. Zeanah, 236–49. New York: Guilford.

Volkmar, Fred R., and Donald J. Cohen. 1985. The experience of infantile autism: A first-person account by Tony W. *Journal of Autism and Developmental Disorders* 15:47–54.

Warren, Frank. 1984. The role of the national society in working with families. In *The effects of autism on the family,* ed. Eric Schopler and Gary B. Mesibov, 99–115. New York: Plenum.

White, B. B., and M. S. White. 1987. Autism from the inside. *Medical Hypotheses* 24:223–29.

Wiebe, Lauren, and Dan Wiebe. N.d. She says, he says: Progress reports from a mixed marriage. *Our Voice* 1, no. 4:15–16.

Williams, Donna. 1992. *Nobody nowhere: The extraordinary autobiography of an autistic.* New York: Times Books.

———. 1994a. Invited commentary: In the real world. *Journal of the Association for Persons with Severe Handicaps* 19:196–99.

———. 1994b. *Somebody somewhere: Breaking free from the world of autism.* New York: Times Books.

———. N.d. About "fighting autism." *Our Voice* 2, no. 1:6–8.

Zatlow, Gerri. 1982. A sister's lament. *Exceptional Parent* 12:50–51.

Zero to Three/National Center for Clinical Infant Programs. 1994. *Diagnostic classification: 0–3: Diagnostic classification of mental health and developmental disorders of infancy and early childhood.* Arlington, Va.: National Center for Clinical Infant Programs.

ADDITIONAL READINGS

Diagnosis of Autism and Related Disorders

Baird, Gillian, Tony Charman, Simon Baron-Cohen, Antony Cox, John Swettenham, Sally Wheelwright, and Auriol Drew. 2000. A screening instrument for autism at 18 months of age: A 6-year follow-up study. *Journal of the Academy for Child and Adolescent Psychiatry* 39: 694–702.

Cohen, Ira L., Vicki Sudhalter, Al Pfadt, Edmund C. Jenkins, W. Ted Brown, and Peter M. Vietze. 1991. Why are autism and fragile-X syndrome associated? Conceptual and methodological issues. *American Journal of Human Genetics* 48:195–202.

Deonna, Thierry W. 1991. Acquired epileptiform aphasia Landau-Kleffner syndrome. *Journal of Clinical Neurophysiology* 8:288–98.

Filipek, Pauline A. et al. 2000. Practice parameter: Screening and diagnosis of autism, report of the quality standards subcommittee of the American Academy of Neurology and the Child Neurology Society, *Neurology* 55: 468–479.

Gillberg, Christopher. 1989. The borderland of autism and Rett syndrome: Five case histories to highlight diagnostic difficulties. *Journal of Autism and Developmental Disorders* 194:545–59.

Klin, Ami, Fred R. Volkmar, Sara S. Sparrow, Domenic V. Cicchetti, and Byron P. Rourke. 1995. Validity and neuropsychological characterization of Asperger Syndrome: Convergence with nonverbal learning disabilities syndrome. *Journal of Child Psychology and Psychiatry* 36:1127–40.

Lehrman, Pinchas, Tally Lehrman-Sagie, and Sara Kivity. 1991. Effect of early corticosteroid therapy for Landau-Kleffner syndrome. *Developmental Medicine and Child Neurology* 33:257–66.

Marescaux, C., E. Hirsch, S. Finck, P. Maquet, E. Schlumberger, F. Sellal, M. N. Metz-Lutz, Y. Alembik, E. Salmon, G. Franck, and D. Kurtz. 1990. Landau-Kleffner syndrome: A pharmacologic study of five cases. *Epilepsia* 31:768–77.

Sawhney, Inder, M. S. Iain, J. A. Robertson, Charles E. Polkey, Colin D. Binnie, and Robert D. C. Elwes. 1995. Multiple subpial transection: A review of 21 cases. *Journal of Neurology, Neurosurgery and Psychiatry* 58:344–49.

Smalley, Susan L., Robert F. Asarnow, and M. Anne Spence. 1988. Autism and genetics: A decade of research. *Archives of General Psychiatry* 45:953–61.

Stefanatos, Gerry A., Warren Grover, and Evan Geller. 1995. Case study: Corticosteroid treatment of language regression in pervasive developmental disorder. *Journal of the American Academy of Child and Adolescent Psychiatry* 34:1107–11.

Szatmari, Peter. 1992. The validity of autistic spectrum disorders: A literature review. *Journal of Autism and Developmental Disorders* 22:583–600.

Developmental Perspectives

Attwood, Tony. 1998. *Asperger's syndrome: A guide for parents and professionals.* London: Jessica Kingsley Publishers.

Dawson, Geraldine, and Arthur Lewy. 1989. Arousal, attention, and the socioemotional impairments of individuals with autism. In *Autism: Nature, diagnosis, and treatment,* ed. Geraldine Dawson, 49–74. New York: Guilford.

Gardner, Howard. 1983. *Frames of mind: The theory of multiple intelligences.* New York: Basic Books.

Greenspan, Stanley I., and Serena Wieder. 1998. *The child with special needs: Encouraging intellectual and emotional growth.* Reading, Mass: Addison Wesley.

Happe, Francesca. 1995. *Autism: An introduction to psychological theory.* Cambridge, Mass.: Harvard University Press.

Schopler, Eric, and Gary B. Mesibov, eds. 1995. *Learning and cognition in autism.* New York: Plenum.

Schopler, Eric, Mary E. Van Bourgondien, and Marie M. Bristol, eds. 1993. *Preschool issues in autism.* New York: Plenum.

Wetherby, Amy M., and Barry M. Prizant, eds. 2000. *Autism spectrum disorders: A transactional developmental perspective.* Baltimore, MD: Paul Brookes.

Behavioral Issues

Koegel, Lynn K., Robert L. Koegel, and Glen Dunlap, eds. 1996. *Positive behavioral support: Including people with difficult behavior in the community.* Baltimore, Md.: Paul Brookes.

Reichle, Joe, and David P. Wacker, eds. 1993. *Communicative alternatives to challenging behavior: Integrating functional assessment and intervention strategies.* Baltimore, Md.: Paul Brookes.

Schopler, Eric, and Gary B. Mesibov, eds. 1994. *Behavioral issues in autism.* New York: Plenum.

Singh, Nirbhay N., ed. 1997. *Prevention and treatment of severe behavior problems: Models and methods in developmental disabilities.* Pacific Grove, Calif.: Brooks/ Cole.

Educational Treatment

Frost, Lori A. and Andrew S. Bondy. 1994. *PECS: The picture exchange communication system: Training manual.* Cherry Hill, N.J.: Pyramid Educational Consultants.

Goldstein, Howard. 1993. Use of peers as communication intervention agents. *Teaching Exceptional Children* 25, no. 2:37–40.

Handleman, Jan S., and Sandra Harris, eds. 2001. *Preschool education programs for children with autism.* 2d ed. Austin, Tex.: PRO-ED.

Harris, Sandra L., Jan S. Handleman, Rita Gordon, Barbara Kristoff, and Felica Fuentes. 1991. Changes in cognitive and language functioning of preschool children with autism. *Journal of Autism and Developmental Disorders* 21:281–90.

New York State Department of Health, Early Intervention Program. 1999. *Clinical practice guideline: Report of the recommendations, autism/pervasive developmental disorders, assessment and intervention for young children (age 0–3 years).* Publication no. 4215. Albany, N.Y.

Quill, Kathleen Ann, ed. 1995. *Teaching children with autism: Strategies to enhance communication and socialization.* New York: Delmar.

Quill, Kathleen Ann. 2000. *Do-watch-listen-say: Social and communication intervention for children with autism.* Baltimore, Md.: Paul Brookes.

Rogers, Sally, and David L. DiLalla. 1991. A comparative study of the effects of a developmentally based instructional model on young children with autism and other disorders of behavior and development. *Topics in Early Childhood Special Education* 11, no. 2:29–47.

Smith, Tristram, Annette D. Groen, and Jacqueline W. Wynn. 2000. Randomized trial of intensive early intervention for children with pervasive developmental disorder. *American Journal on Mental Retardation* 105:269–85.

Watson, Linda R., Catherine Lord, Bruce Schaffer, and Eric Schopler. 1989. *Teaching spontaneous communication to autistic and developmentally handicapped children.* Austin,Tex.: PRO-ED.

Facilitated Communication

Biklen, Douglas. 1990. Communication unbound: Autism and praxis. *Harvard Educational Review* 60:291–314.

———. 1993. *Communication unbound: How facilitated communication is challenging traditional views of autism and ability/disability.* New York: Teachers College Press.

Green, Gina, and Howard C. Shane. 1994. Science, reason, and facilitated communication. *Journal of the Association for the Severely Handicapped* 19:151–71.

Medical Perspectives

Baker, Sidney M., and Jon Pangborn. 1996. *Clinical assessment options for children with autism and related disorders: A biomedical approach.* San Diego, Calif.: Autism Research Institute.

Cook, Edwin H., and Bennett L. Leventhal. 1995. Pediatric psychopharmacology II: Autistic disorder and other pervasive developmental disorders. *Child and Adolescent Psychiatric Clinics of North America* 4:381–99.

McDougle, Christopher J., Lawrence H. Price, and Fred R. Volkmar. 1994. Recent advances in the pharmacotherapy of autism and related conditions. *Child and Adolescent Psychiatric Clinics of North America* 3:71–90.

Thatcher, Robert W., G. Reid Lyon, Judith Rumsey, and Norman Krasnegor, eds. 1996. *Developmental neuroimaging: Mapping the development of brain and behavior.* San Diego, Calif.: Academic Press.

Parental Perspectives

Hamilton, Lynn M. 2000. *Facing autism: Giving parents reasons for hope and guidance for help.* Colorado Springs: Waterbrook.

Seroussi, Karyn. 2000. *Unraveling the mystery of autism and pervasive developmental disorder: A mother's story of research and recovery.* New York: Simon and Schuster.

Index

abuse: physical, 66–67, 151; self-, 47–49, 77, 86; sexual, 151. *See also* self-injurious behavior

accommodation: combined with adaptation, 108; in TEACCH, 104

ACTH drug, 15, 16

adaptive behavior, special education and, 88, 108

adolescence, 54–62, 181; follow-up studies, 161–64, 170; medication, 177; TEACCH and, 106

adulthood, 54–62, 162–71; follow-up studies, 162–65, 170; insider descriptions, 21–32, 183–86; jobs, 58, 59–60, 106, 183; medication, 177; near-normal functioning, 82; "person-centered planning," 181–83; and recovery, 82–83, 162–71; services, 106, 181

advocacy, 119–34, 178–83. *See also* parent groups

Advocate, 13

affect. *See* emotions

African-American woman, at Westchester conference, 75, 76, 80–81, 133

age: of onset, 8–9. *See also* developmental patterns; *specific age groups*

aggression: in adolescence, 55; in adulthood, 61; FC and, 152; medication for, 86, 177; restraint holds and, 101. *See also* self-injurious behavior

AIT. *See* auditory integration training

alien experiences, 29–32. *See also* differentness

alternative treatment, 85–86, 135–54; AIT, 65, 85, 86, 140–42, 169; dietary, 85, 138–39, 142; FC, 144–48, 149–53; sensory integration therapy, 85, 142–44; vitamin therapy, 85, 86, 138

American Psychiatric Association, 4–5

American Psychologist, 144–45, 151–52

amygdala, 175

Anderson, Stephen R., 88

ANI (Autism Network International), 183–84, 185

Anthropologist on Mars. See Sacks, Oliver

anticonvulsant medications, 16

antifungal diets, 139

207

repetition: autistic, 6, 17, 23, 38. *See also* rituals; stereotyped behaviors
research, 20–21, 137; into AIT, 141–42; and antifungal treatments, 139; biomedical, 174–76, 177–78; and dietary treatment, 139; on educational treatment, 87, 112, 117–18; on facilitated communication, 151–52; on immune system functioning, 139–40; on movement 148–49, 154; outcome data, 117–18, 162–65; parents behind, 177–78; on sensory integration therapy, 142–44; on vitamins, 138
resistance to change, 16, 23. *See also* predictability
respite care services, 70, 71
responding to multiple cues, pivotal behavior, 114, 115
Rett syndrome / Rett's disorder, 7
Rimland, Bernard, 136–38, 140, 141, 166
rituals, 17, 23, 55, 101, 177. *See also* play; stereotyped behaviors
Rogers, Sally, 148, 178
rote learning, in behavioral approaches, 98–99
Rutgers University, Douglass Developmental Disabilities Center, 87, 96–97, 98
Rutter, Michael, 52, 159

Sacks, Oliver, *Anthropologist on Mars:* autistic family, 13; Grandin case study, 4, 28, 30, 160, 185–86; married couple with Asperger's syndrome, 184
sameness. *See* predictability
Scariano, Margaret M., 20, 24, 25
schizoid personality, vs. Asperger's syndrome, 12
Schlachter, Mimi, 53
Schloss, Hadassah M., 121
school districts, 121–34. *See also* education; inclusion; special education
Schopler, Eric, 104, 105
Schreibman, Laura, 114
Schulze, Craig, 5, 8–9, 11, 64, 66, 83
Seaver Center for Autism Research and Treatment, 139–40
seizures, 15, 48, 55. *See also* epilepsy
self-injurious behavior, 47–49, 55, 77, 86, 97
self-management, pivotal behavior, 114, 115–16
self-stimulating behaviors, 38, 77, 89. *See also* stereotyped behaviors
sensory functioning: AIT and, 140–42; infants and, 36–38; insider descriptions of,

26–27; in sensory integration therapy, 142–44
sensory integration therapy, 85, 113, 142–44
serotonin dysfunctions, 48, 138, 176
services. *See* education; treatment
sexual abuse, 151
"shadow," 132
Shaw, William, 139
siblings, of autistic children, 7, 64, 65, 67–68, 70
Siblings of Children with Autism (Harris), 68
Siege (Park), 83
sign language, 109, 154
Sinclair, Jim, 183; alien experience, 30; connection difficulties, 28, 29; poem, 32; speech and language difficulties, 25–26, 27–28
Smith, Tristram, 161
social interaction, 5, 23–25, 38; of autistic adults, 20, 29–30, 60–61, 159, 183–85; conversations, 50, 57–58, 160; eye contact, 35, 36, 37, 89; FC and, 152–53; fragile X syndrome and, 18; by infants, 35–37; marriages, 184–85; in middle childhood, 50–52; by preschoolers, 44, 46–47; theory of mind in, 50–52; by toddlers, 44; treatment and, 89–90, 98. *See also* communication; families; friendships; people; reciprocal interaction
social referencing, 35–36
Son Rise (Kaufman), 166
Son Rise: The Miracle Continues (Kaufman), 166
Son-Rise program, 167–69
Sound of a Miracle (Stehli), 8, 140–41
spatial intelligence, 54
special abilities, of autistic individuals, 9, 43–44, 52–54, 55–56, 61–62
special education, 86–118, 123–24, 173–74, 178–81. *See also* behavioral approaches; education; federal special education laws; one-to-one teaching; treatment
speech: of autistic adults, 5, 6, 25–26, 60–61; echoing of, 41–42; FC and, 146, 147; Landau-Kleffner syndrome and, 14–15, 16; in middle childhood, 50; and motor disorders, 40, 149; outcome data and, 165; PECS training and, 108–9; by preschoolers, 38–43; therapy, 25–26, 96–97, 113. *See also* communication; language
Squeeze Machine, 143
Staten Island, and public funding for behavioral programs, 125–26, 133
Stefanatos, Gerry, 14, 16

Compositor: Maple-Vail Manufacturing Group
Text: Palatino
Display: Snell Roundhand Script and Bauer Bodoni
Printer and binder: Maple-Vail Manufacturing Group